Quantum Healing

Published April 09, 2017 by HetHeru AnkhBaRa

Printed in the United States of America.

ISBN-13: 978-1545124420
ISBN-10: 1545124426

HEALING BLUE LOTUS
HETHERU ANKHBARA
P.O. BOX 814
CENTRAL ISLIP, N.Y. 11722
healingbluelotus.com
718.314.4492

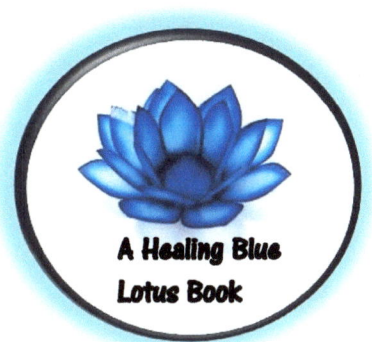

A Healing Blue

Lotus Book

To:

From: Author

The future is NOW.

LOVE. HEAL. THRIVE!

Love,

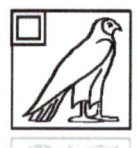

———————————————

HetHeru AnkhBaRa

Dedicated

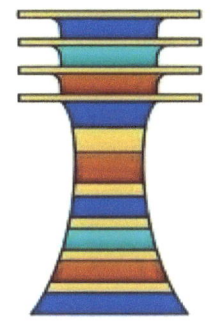

I dedicate this book

to our

beloved

Dr. Sebi.

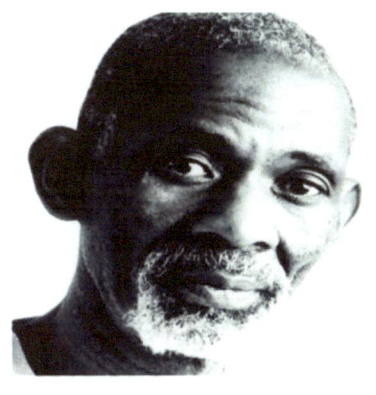

Love and gratitude.

- HetHeru AnkhBaRa

Healing Blue Lotus

Presents

The Quantum Body Examiner

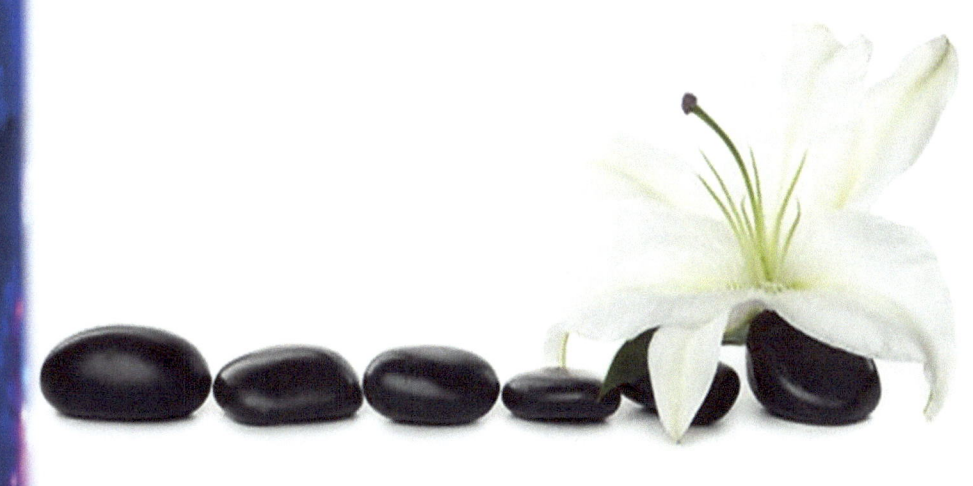

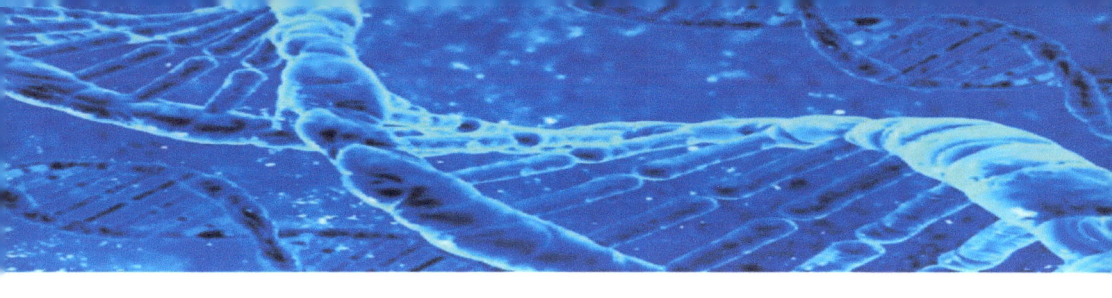

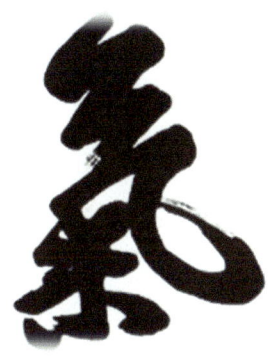

Qi/Chi according to Traditional Chinese Medicine includes information, vibration, frequency, and energy. Qi/Chi can be manipulated with thought as in self-healing or distant healing or with a tool, such as an acupuncture needle or an Omega wand. It is not the needle or the wand that heals, but the Qi/Chi that awakens the body's own healing energy to transform the state of disharmony/disease.

Let's take it to the roots.

Chi.

Its roots can be traced back to AFRICA.

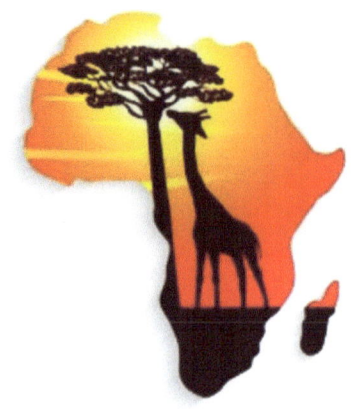

The Kemetyu (Ancient Egyptians)

called it Sekhem.

Keep in mind that:

" Nothing rests; everything moves; everything vibrates."

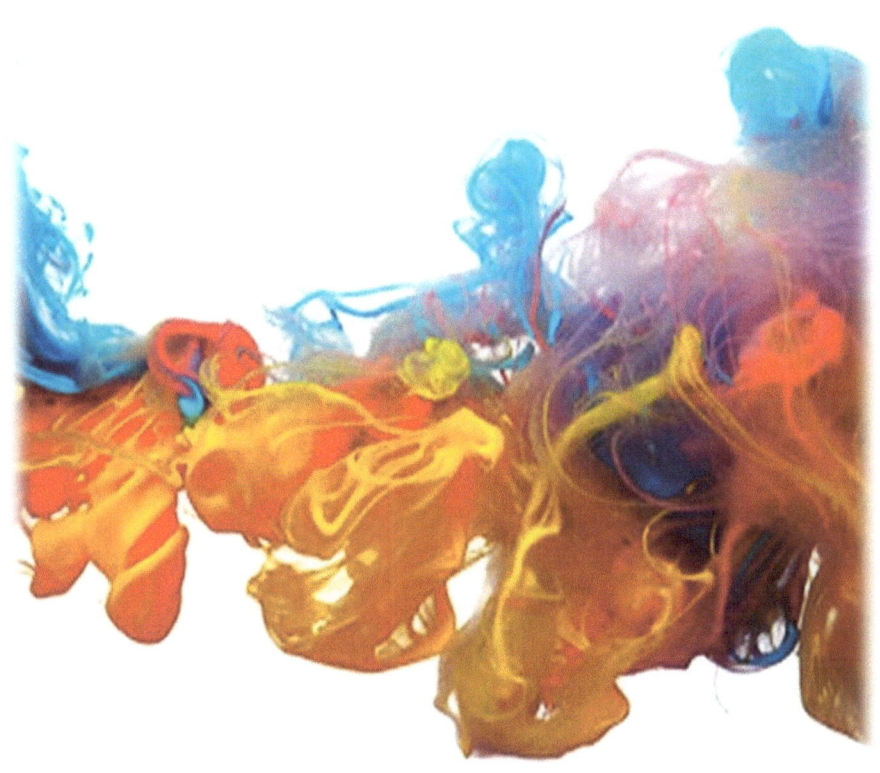

- Jhuty

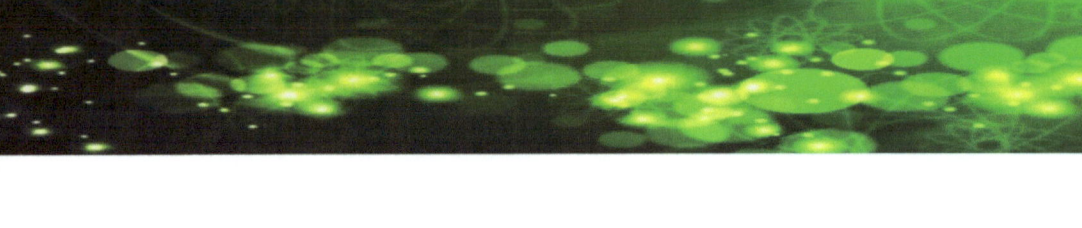

<u>The whole universe is energy, and each basic element of the atomic chart consists of energy at different rates of vibration.</u>

- The difference between any two elements is the difference in both atomic structure and vibrational rates. On the physical plane, you are vibrating at a rate that is different than the rate on the spiritual plane. There is a frequency or vibration of energy that fills the universe. This energy is essential to all living cells, humans, plants, and animals.

- We utilize this energy with our minds. Every thought is transmitted by this energy, and every aspect of physical life depends on this basic energy or power of the universe.

- Good energy is very important for spiritual growth, and spiritual growth is our ultimate purpose and reason for being alive on this physical plane called Earth. Each individual must learn how to utilize this energy for spiritual growth and development. If we use this energy constructively we can raise our level of consciousness, and vibrational rate or frequency, remember, every individual has a different rate of vibration. Raise your vibration baby!

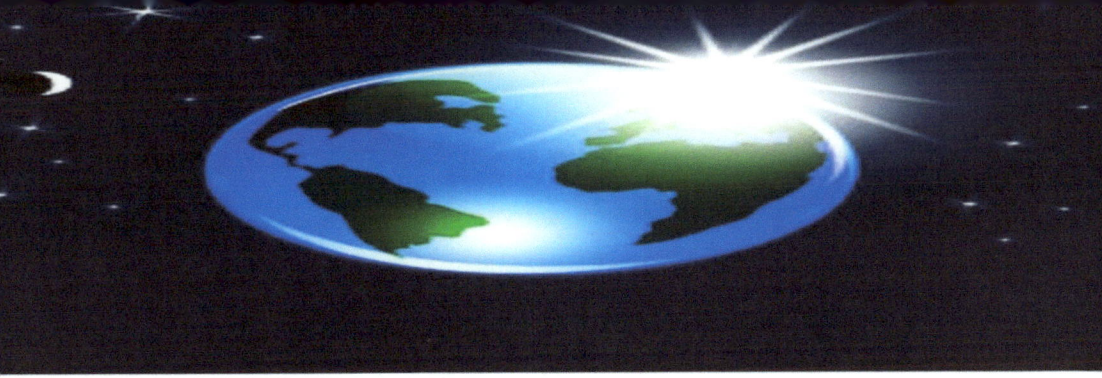

- All of man's earthly problems are created by his thoughts. What we project from our mind in the form of thoughts, we create.

- <u>Spiritual growth requires infinite LOVE in your HEART, and the elimination of disagreeable thoughts, which can dissipate the Sekhem, the life force energy.</u>

- The Kemeyu taught that the Ethereal Substance is very elastic, and pervades universal space in all directions, serving as a medium of transmission of waves of vibratory energy, such as heat, light, electricity, magnetism, etc. The teachings are that the Ethereal Substance is a connecting link between the forms of vibratory energy known as "Matter" on the one hand, and "Energy or Force" on the other; and also, that Ethereal Substance manifests a degree of vibration, at a rate entirely all its own.

The Quantum Medicine Phenomenal

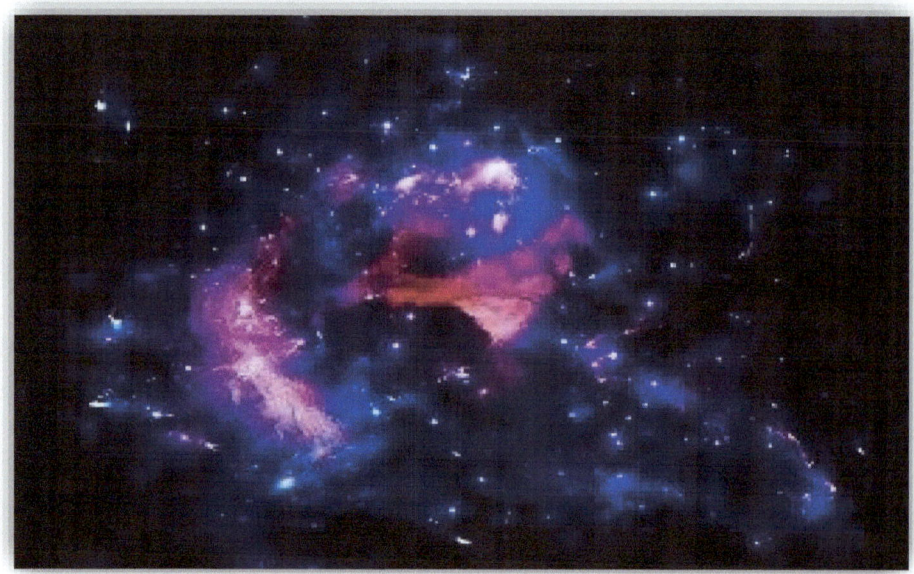

Quantum Medicine:

Quantum Medicine is the science of healing, and it mirrors Chinese Medicine in the use of energy to bring the body back to a state of balance and harmony. In all-natural medicine such as Chinese Medicine, Ayurveda Medicine, Native American, Homeopathy and a host of other natural healing alternative medicines, energy is used. Quantum Medicine is an informational medicine. It is the science of consciousness and information in healing and provides a broad spectrum of multi-disciplines and protocols to address the complexities of chronic illness and pain.

Western Medicine

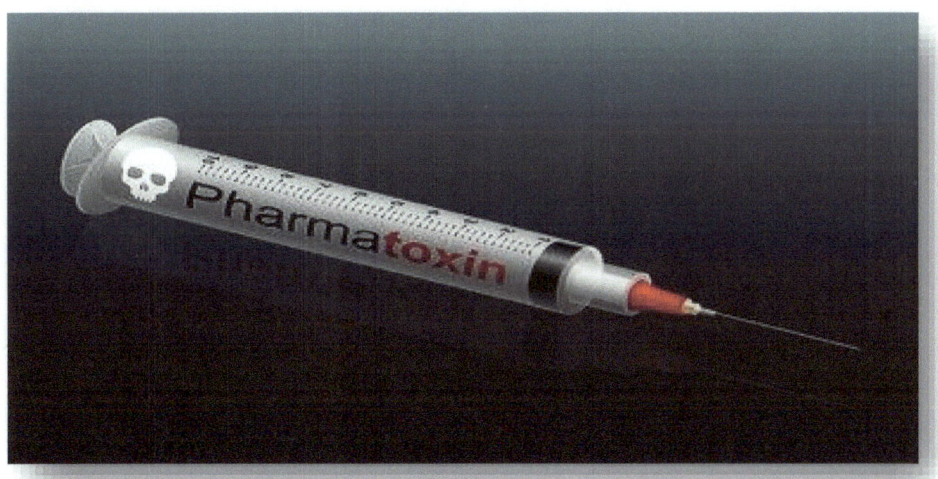

Western medicine has a different view based on counting and measuring. It has a different view of reality, too. It does not recognize the phenomenon of energy, information, belief, thought, intention, Qi or energy healing, therefore, when such events occur or are observed it is called the Placebo Effect.

Consider what the Placebo Effect means in Western Medicine. When the client or patient believes a substance to have medicinal value or beliefs in the doctor; the authority that prescribes it yet receives the same benefit from a sugar pill containing no active ingredient it is called the Placebo Effect.

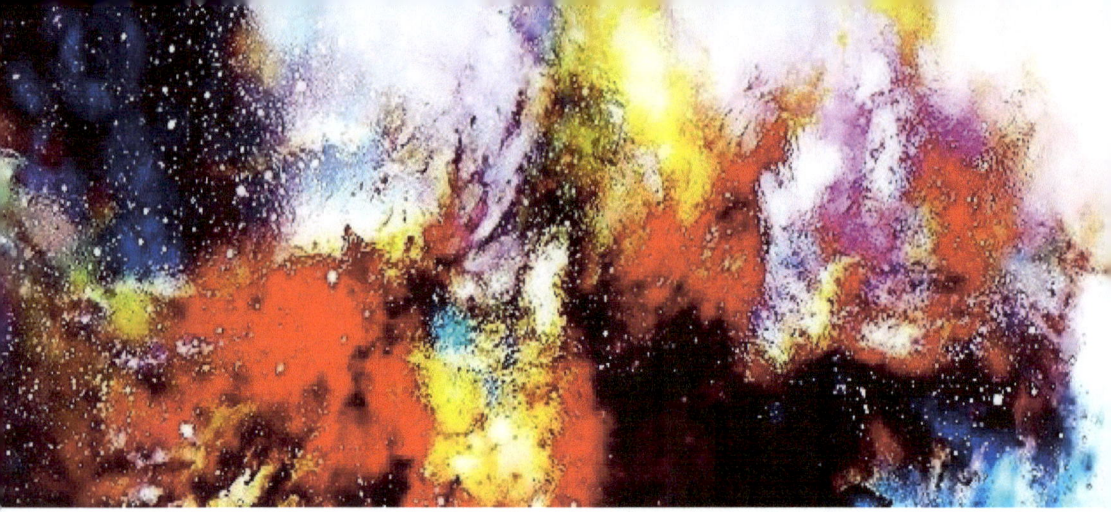

The Body is An Energy Field

The body is an energy field and in a constant state of change. Most ailments begin from a change in energy. Energy is affected by beliefs, thought, emotions, attitude, what we eat and drink, the amount of exercise or lack thereof, stress, work, rest habits and lifestyles, as well as changes in weather and environment.

Chinese Medicine and Energy Medicines use a wide spectrum of disciplines to address disharmony, stagnation, illness, and pain. Acupuncture is one of the most well-known and uses a needle to manipulate Qi/Chi or energy. The needle is a tool used to manipulate and direct the energy flow in the body along the meridians. The body's own Qi/Chi or vital energy does the work necessary to balance, harmonize and strengthen, to repair itself.

Quantum Taoist Medicine and Acupuncture

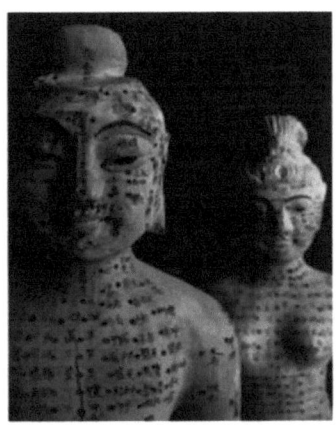

Quantum Chinese (Taoist philosophy) Medicine promotes the study of Qi, Yin and Yang, and the Cycle of the Four Seasons of life in-depth to facilitate the understanding of human psychology and the appropriate use of herbs, formulas, and homeopathic remedies. A description of the "anatomy of meridians" is presented to enable the personalization of the meridians and to understand the genesis of disharmony leading to disease from an energetic point of view.

The integration of acupuncture with advanced concepts in Quantum biofeedback is included, as well as an understanding of the "marvelous vessels" and their correlation with the Five Organ Systems. The acupuncture meridians and the concepts of the "atomic heart" and the "creation yin-yang," are an integral part of the understanding in the multiple relationships between Qi/Chi, the meridians and the viscera.

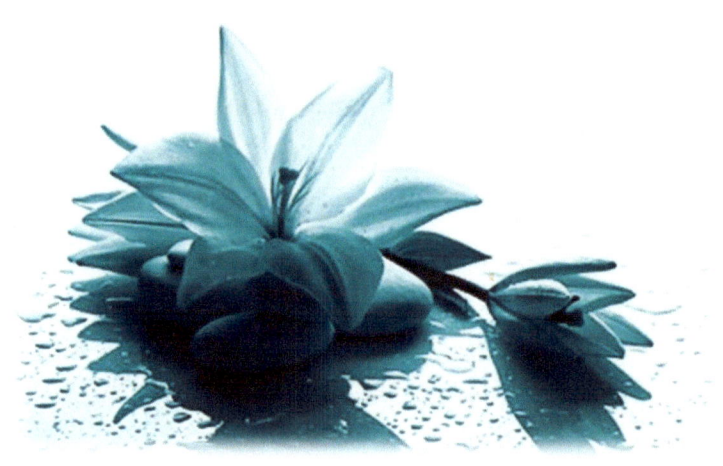

The future is **NOW.**

Prepare thyself; for I am going to put the power of better health in your HANDS!

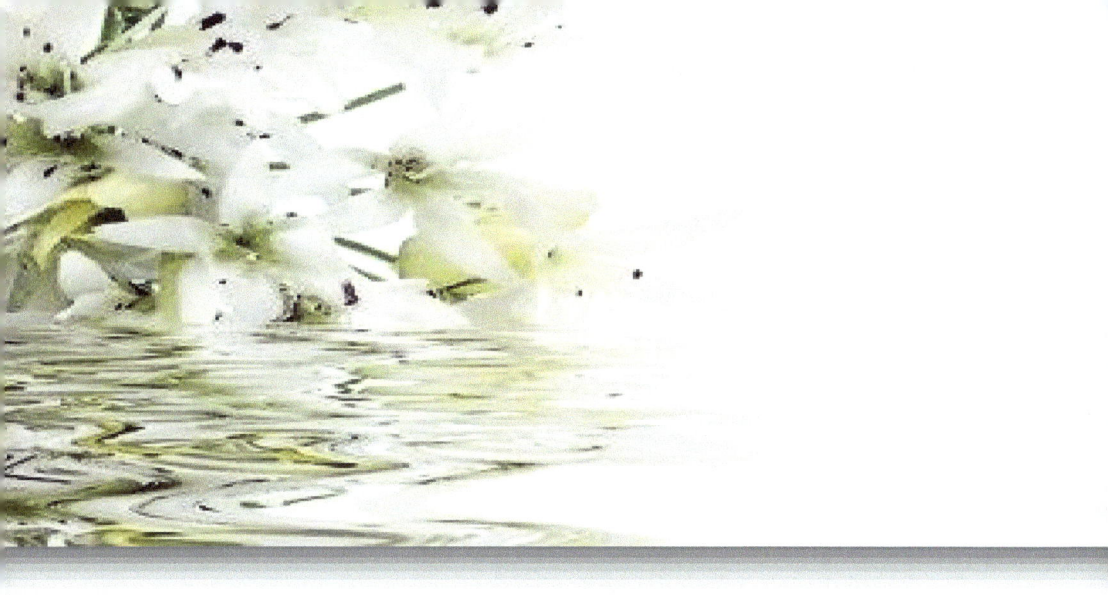

The Quantum Body Examiner, A High-Tech Innovation That Combines the Best of Medicine, Bio-Informatics, Electrical Engineering and Other Sciences.

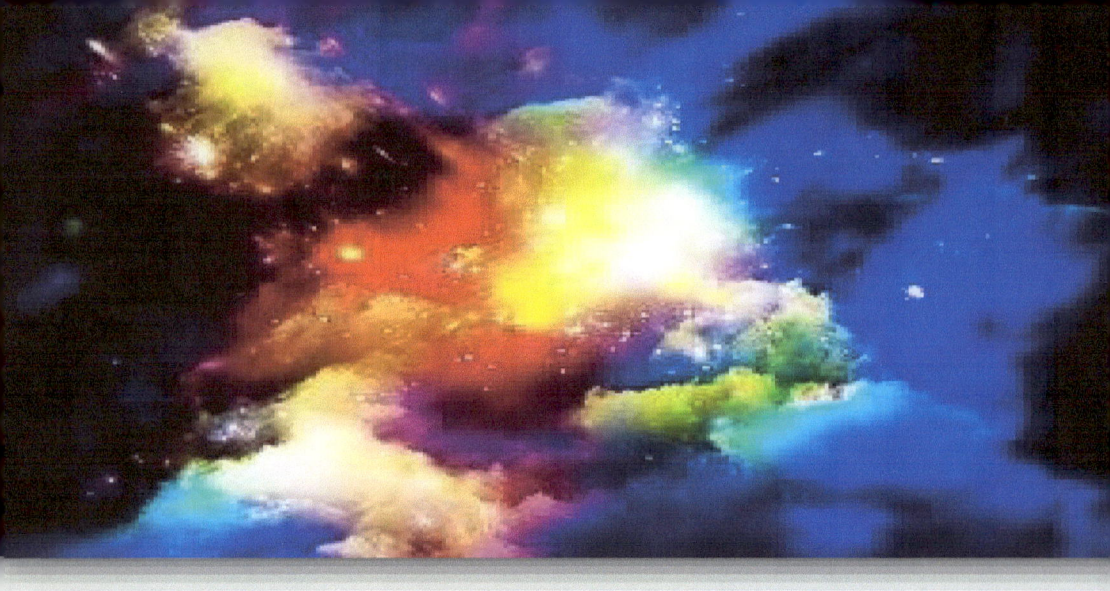

The Quantum Body Examiner will analyze your condition or the condition of your patient/client's health without blood analysis or radiography. No radiation. No blood is drawn. No kidding!

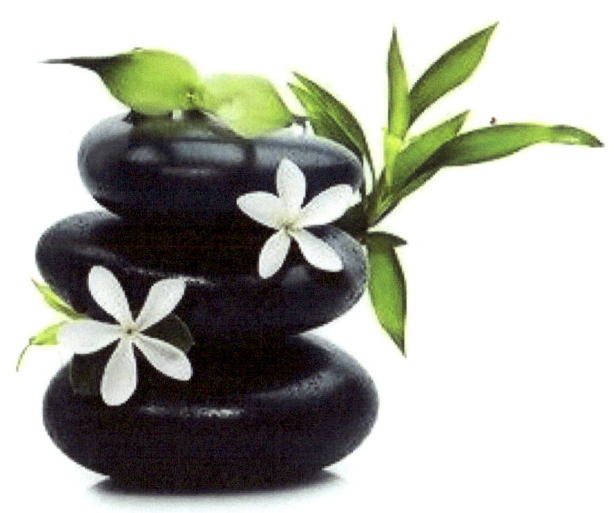

How Does the Quantum Body Examiner work?

The Quantum Body Examiner uses frequency technology. It is a fashionable and an easy to carry devise. The Quantum Body Examiner requires a connection to a computer/laptop. Followed by a fast and simple software installation.

No More Guesswork...
First Target the Cause...
Stop Treating the Symptoms.

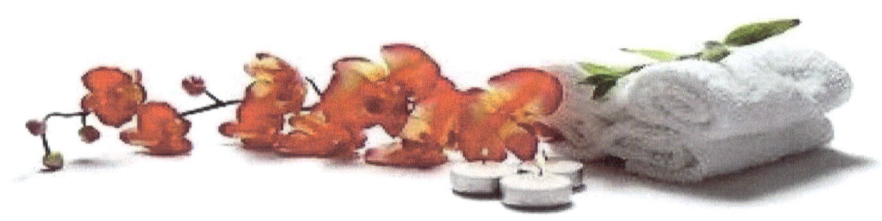

The Quantum Body Examiner comes with a manual and all tools necessary to get you started right away. Besides, it is super easy!

Ask your patient/client to remove all electronic devices. They may sit or lay down. Please ask them to RELAX and BREATH. Kindly, ask them not to speak while they are being scanned. Place the sensor stick in their hand (it does not matter which hand is used, however; I prefer the left hand.)

Simply by having your patient/client hold the sensor in the palm of their hand, a health data will be collected within about three minutes from various body parts. This advanced electronic system collects the weak magnetic field of human cells for scientific analysis and compares each organ with the referenced database; thereby analyzing and determining a person's health status and main problems and putting forward standard prevention recommendations.

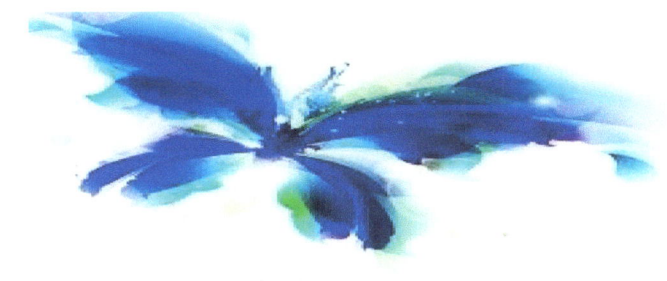

The analysis is non-invasive and will tell you the condition of your health or your patient/client's health without blood analysis or radiation. The Quantum Body Examiner will quickly scan your patient/client. Before you know it, he or she will be done.

The Quantum Body Examiner runs about 60 thousand waves of frequency; through every cell of the body. The Quantum Body Examiner reads the magnetic field of the patient/client. It detects the imbalances; deficiencies and abnormalities of the cells. It then interprets the data and provides a full report.

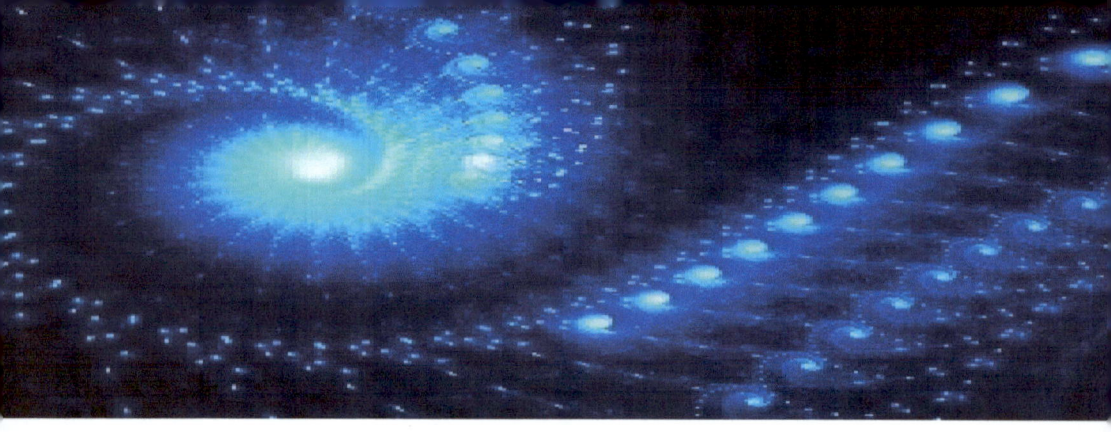

The report includes:

1: CARDIOVASCULAR AND CEREBROVASCULAR

2: GASTROINTESTINAL FUNCTION

3: LIVER FUNCTION

4: GALLBLADDER FUNCTION

5: PANCREATIC FUNCTION

6: KIDNEY FUNCTION

7: LUNG FUNCTION

8: BRAIN NERVE

9: BONE DISEASE

10: BONE MINERAL DENSITY

11: RHEUMATOID BONE DISEASE

12: BONE GROWTH INDEX

13: BLOOD SUGAR

14: TRACE ELEMENT

15: VITAMIN

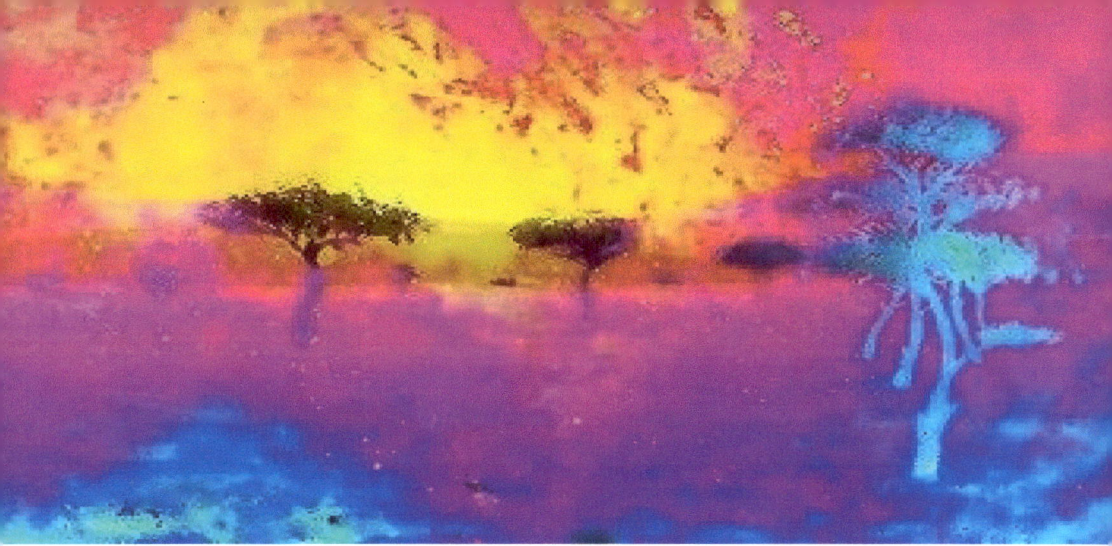

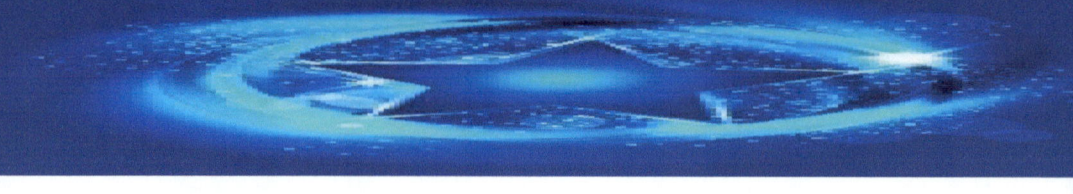

33: PROSTATE (MALE)

34: MALE SEXUAL FUNCTION (MALE)

35: SPERM AND SEMEN (MALE)

36: ELEMENT OF HUMAN

37: GYNECOLOGY (FEMALE)

38: MENSTRUAL CYCLE (FEMALE)

39: BREAST (FEMALE)

40: ADHD (KIDS)

41：TRACE ELEMENT（KIDS）

42：VITAMIN（KIDS）

43：AMINO ACID（KIDS）

44：COENZYME（KIDS）

45: COMPREHENSIVE REPORT CARD

THERE ARE 5 REPORTS EXCLUSIVELY FOR CHILDREN UNDER 10 YEARS OLD. THIS REPORT WILL *ONLY* SHOW FOR CHILDREN UNDER 10 YEARS OF AGE.

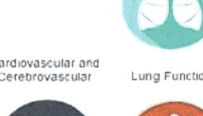 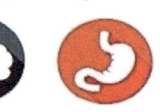 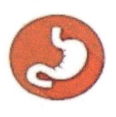  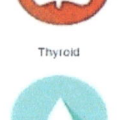 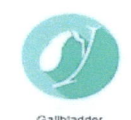 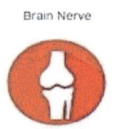 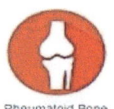  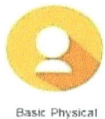 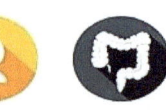

Cardiovascular and Cerebrovascular   Lung Function   Liver Function   Prostate   Brain Nerve   Basic Physical Quality   Large Intestine Function

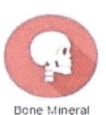 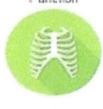 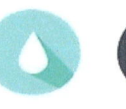    

Kidney Function   Gastrointestinal Function   Thyroid   Gallbladder Function   Rheumatoid Bone Disease   Pancreatic Function   Gynecology

Bone Mineral Density   Bone Disease   Blood Sugar   Trace Element   Male Sexual Function   ADHD   skin

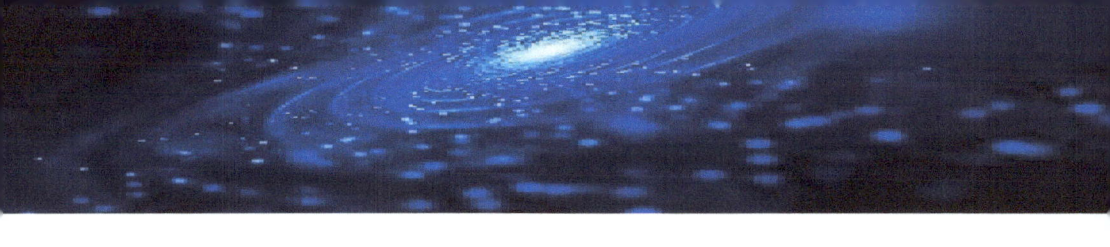

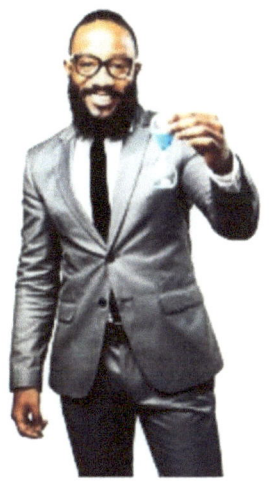

This Means

No More Waiting

For Test Results. Sweet!

The Quantum Body Examiner determines the current health of the organs and predicts their wellbeing for the future.

It helps to uncover the onset of major diseases, which can assist in early treatment and maintenance.

The Quantum Body Examiner is an essential key to excellent health.

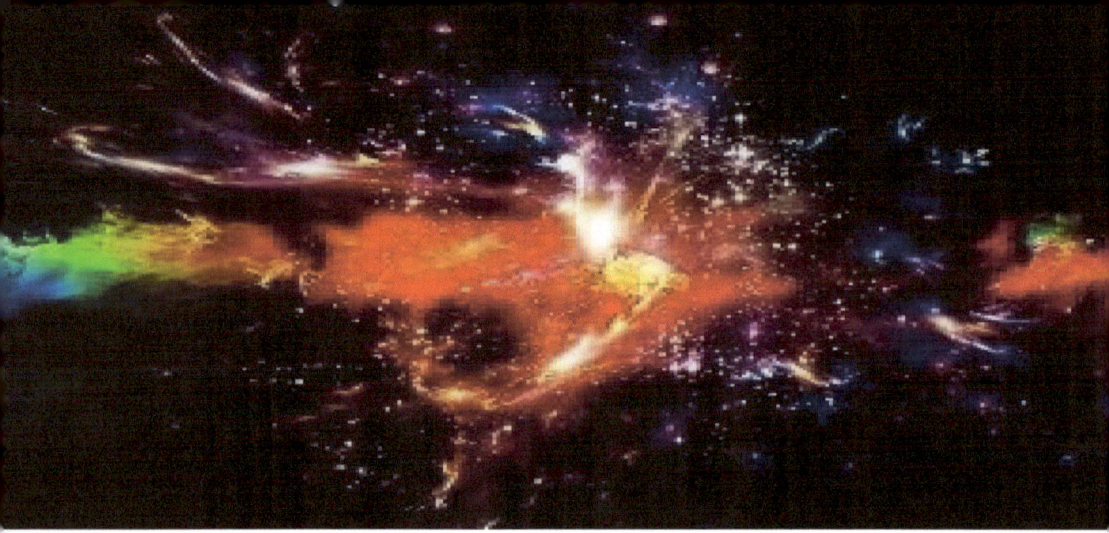

The Quantum Body Examiner replaces the need for ultrasonic, nuclear magnetic resonance and radiography for diagnosing various health related conditions. The Quantum Body Examiner offers a new advantage in the field of material analysis. It has been shown that the applicability of such an analyzer exceeds the range of tissue analysis and other medical applications.

The machine can function in 2 languages English and Spanish.

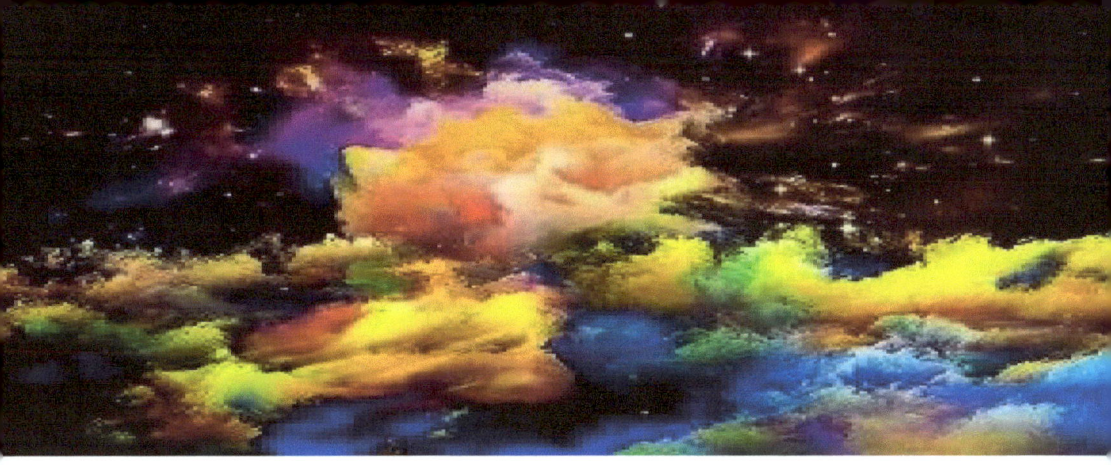

<u>The Quantum Body Examiner Principle of Analysis:</u>

The Human body is an aggregate of numerous cells, which continuously grow develop, split, regenerate and die. By splitting up, cells renew themselves.

For adults, about 25 million cells are splitting up every second. Blood cells are constantly renewing at a rate of about 100 million per minute. In the process of cellular split-up and renewal, the charge bodies of nucleus and extranuclear electrons as the basis unit of a cell are moving and changing ceaselessly at a high speed as well, as emitting electromagnetic waves without interruption. The signals of electromagnetic waves emitted by human bodies represent the specific condition of the human body, and therefore, different signals of electromagnetic waves will be emitted by the conditions of good health or disease.

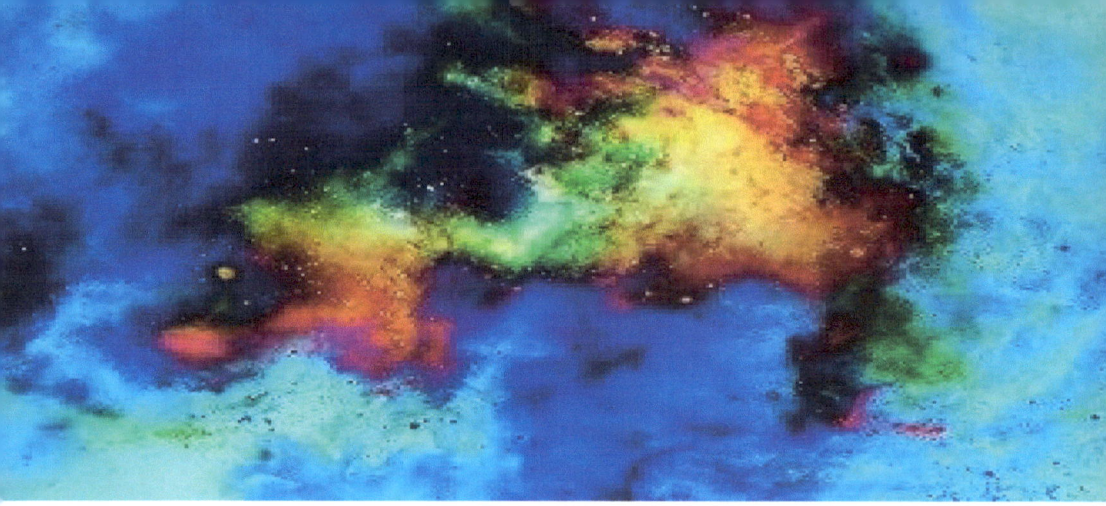

Health conditions can easily be analyzed if such specific electromagnetic wave signals can be examined. The Quantum Body Examiner is a new instrument to analyze such phenomenon.

The weak magnetic frequency and energy of the human body are collected by holding the sensor, and after amplification by the instrument and treatment by the built-in micro-processor, the data are compared with the standard quantum resonance spectrum of diseases, nutrition and other indicators incorporated in the instrument to judge whether the sample waveforms are irregular using the Fourier approach.

Therefore, analysis and judgment can be made on the health condition of the patient/ client based on the result of waveform analysis, as well as standard protective and curative proposals.

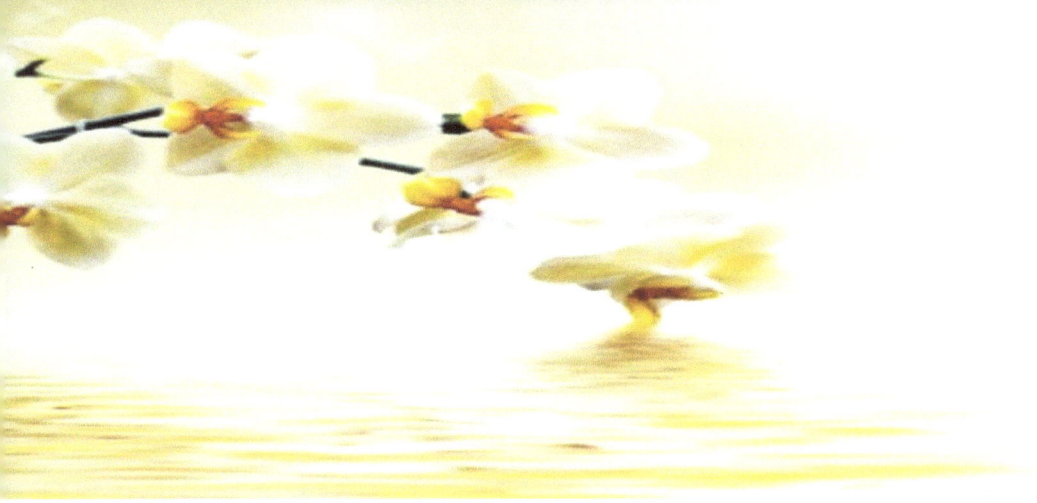

The Quantum Body Examiner comes with Transcutaneous Electrical Nerve Stimulation Therapy (TENS).

TENS, or Transcutaneous Electrical Nerve Stimulation, is a non-invasive, drug free method to control pain by sending tiny electrical impulses through the skin. These impulses stimulate the nerves which send pain blocking signals to the brain. In many cases, this stimulation will greatly reduce or eliminate pain. TENS therapy is used to treat acute and chronic back pain, Sciatic Nerve Pain relief, muscular and disc syndromes, arthritis, shoulder pain, and many other painful conditions.

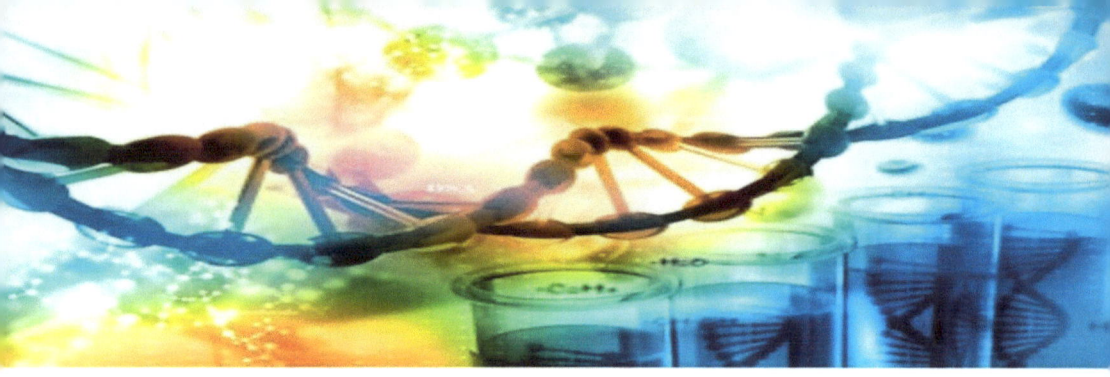

Features:

- Easy to operate, stylish design, and comfortable.

- It must be connected to a computer or laptop.

- It comes with diagnosis and therapy system.

- It comes with automatic treatment.

- Ear and hands acupuncture points stimulation.

- Chinese Medicine Meridian Theory combined with Modern Medical Technology.

- No bleeding or bruise. No side effects.

- The treatment time is short, and there is no need take time off. It will not affect your normal life and work.

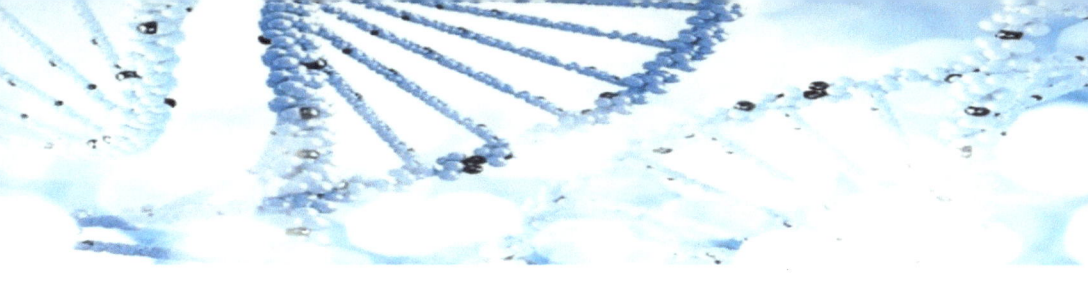

- The system database is based on stern health statistic and built by a large number clinical authentication.

- Speed: Multiple indicators of your health can be obtained within minutes. This analysis method is designed to save you time and money.

- Accuracy: The database of the analysis system has been established with scientific methods. It has been proven to be accurate in a large number of clinical cases.

- The function is non-invasive and painless, the analysis will tell you the condition of your patients/client's health without hemanalysis or radiography.
- Through using this health instrument, a health check can be made anytime and anywhere. It is convenient and easy to use.

<u>Disclaimer: The Quantum Body Examiner does not claim to cure or treat any disease or injury. It assists your body to re-balance it's bio-energy fields and stimulates the body for self-detoxification. The body's organs will function better with a healthy-body.</u>

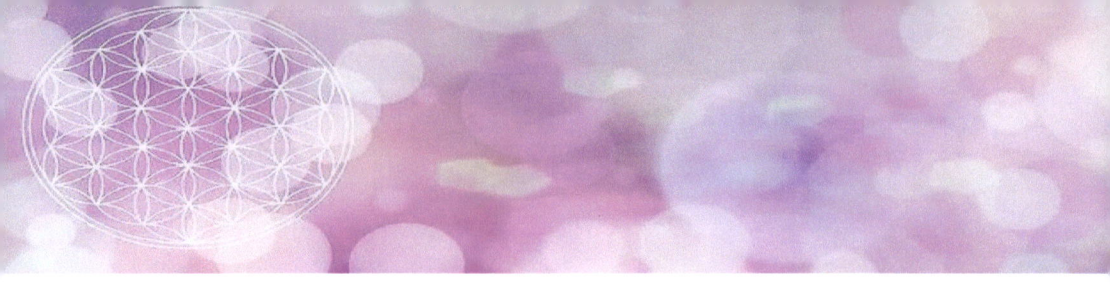

The Quantum Body Examiner Machine

A.K.A. Quantum Resonance Magnetic Analyzer, with therapy function.

We are very proud to offer authentic and certified Quantum machines. Our Quantum Body Examiner machine is a Rockstar!

The Quantum Body Examiner Package includes:

- **Main Body (Include the box) × 1**
- **Detecting handle × 1**
- **Software CD × 1**
- **USB Soft dog × 1**
- **USB Cable × 1**
- **Instruction Manual × 1**
- **Massager Slipper × 1**
- **TENS Pads (TENS: Transcutaneous Electrical Nerve Stimulation) × 2**
- **Ear tester × 2**
- **Hand tester × 2**

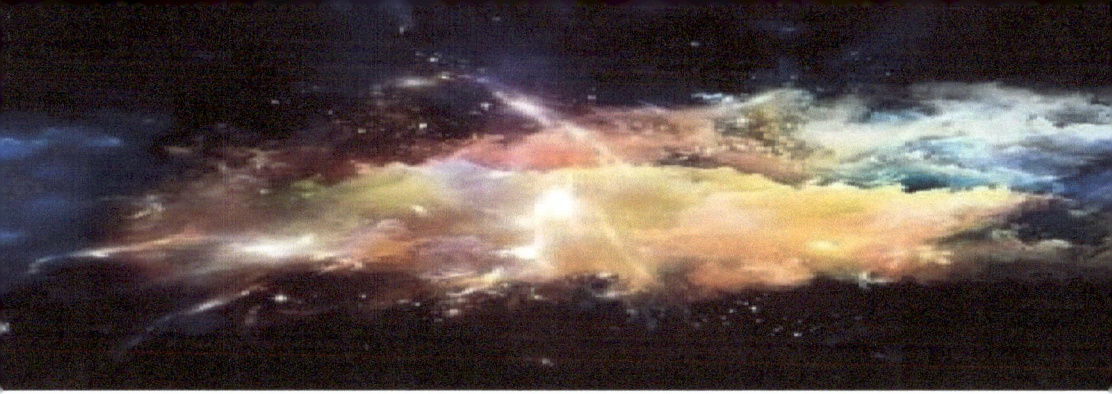

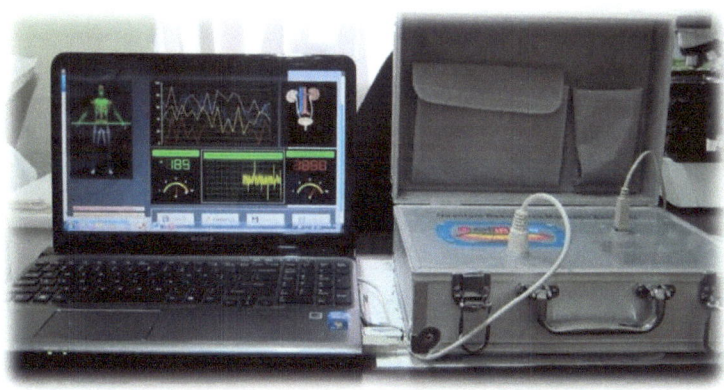

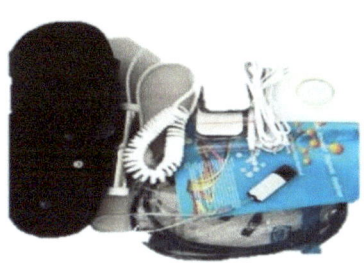

**Operating system:
Windows 98 / SE / ME /
2000 / XP / VISTA / 7 / 8/10**

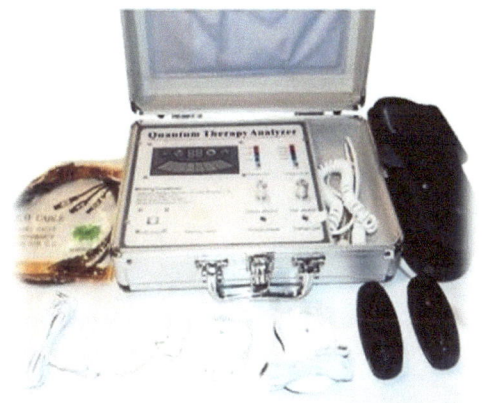

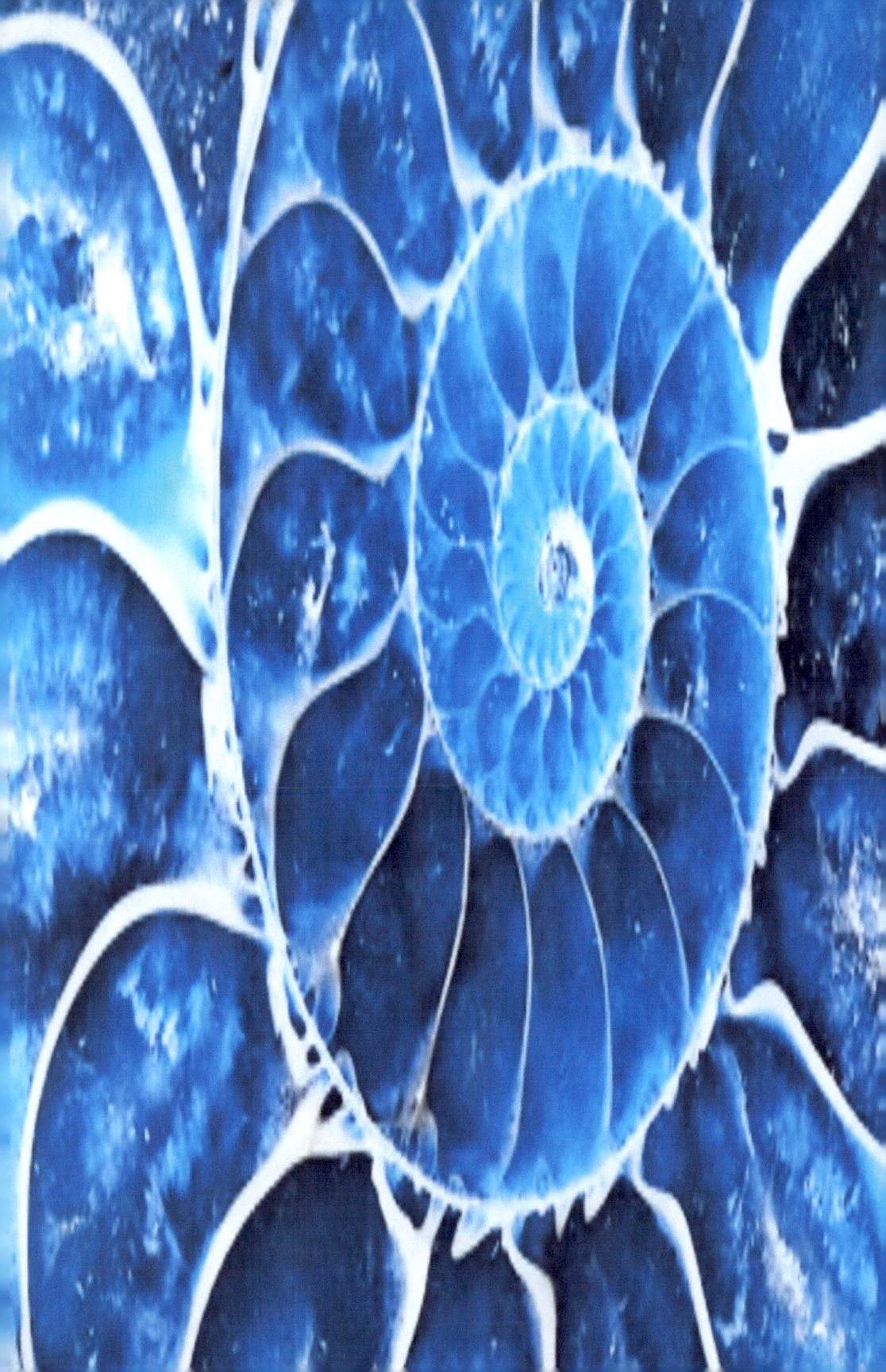

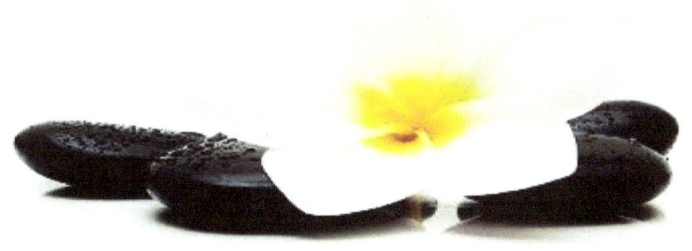

The Quantum Body Examiner Retail Price List

Name   Price

NEW

Quantum Body Examiner, For Your Home Or Office………………...only $249

Wholesale prices are available.

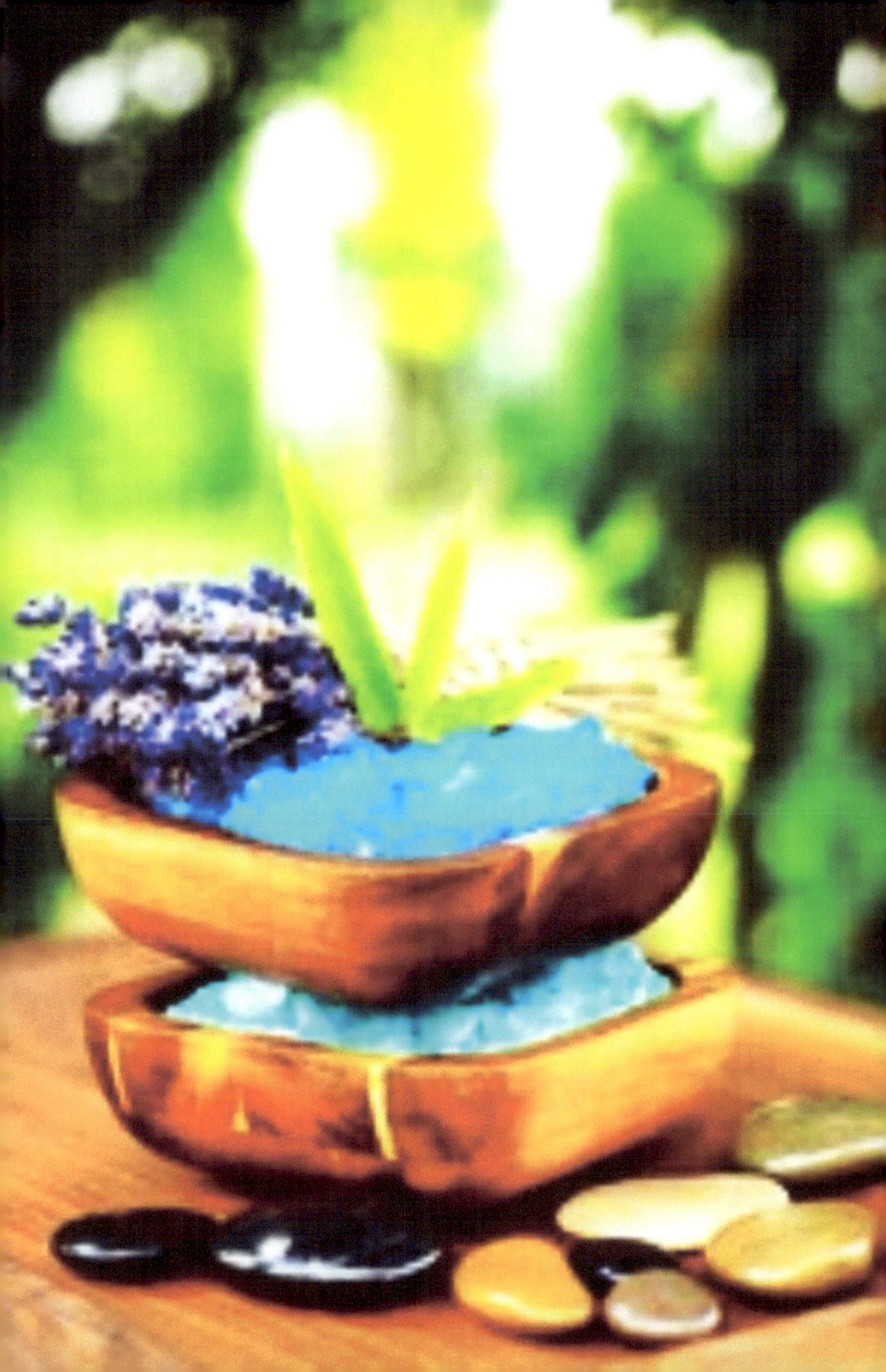

Time to cuddle up with a good book.

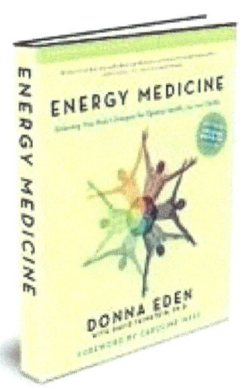

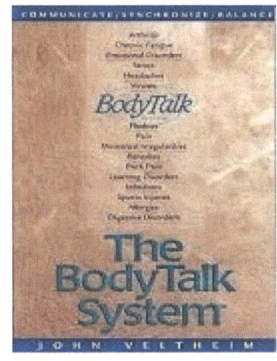

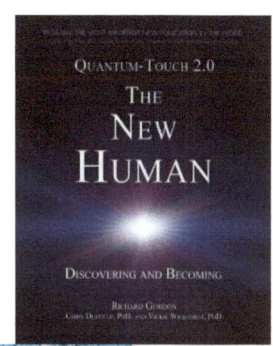

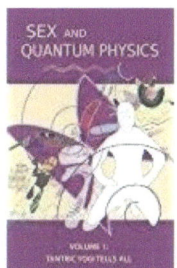

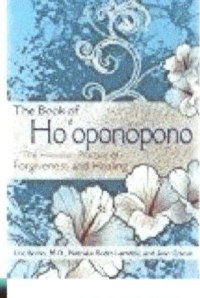

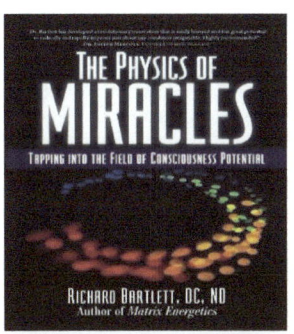

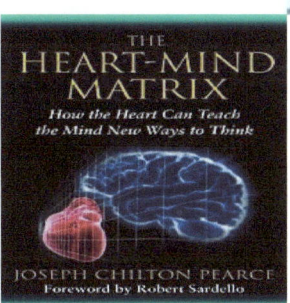

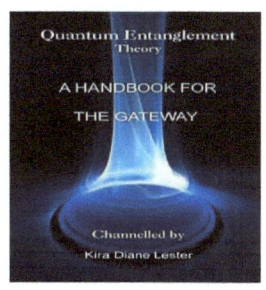

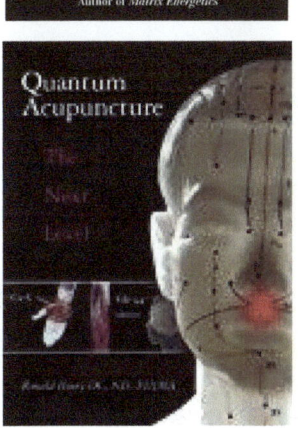

Interesting related books, just to name a few...

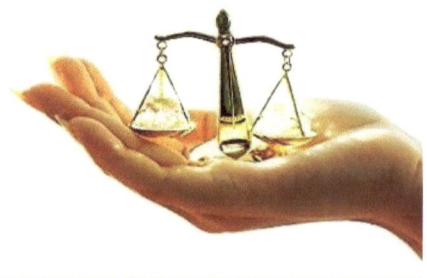

LAWS GOVERNING ENERGY MEDICINE PRACTITIONERS

LINNIE THOMAS

AUTHOR OF THE AWARD WINNING
ENCYCLOPEDIA OF ENERGY MEDICINE

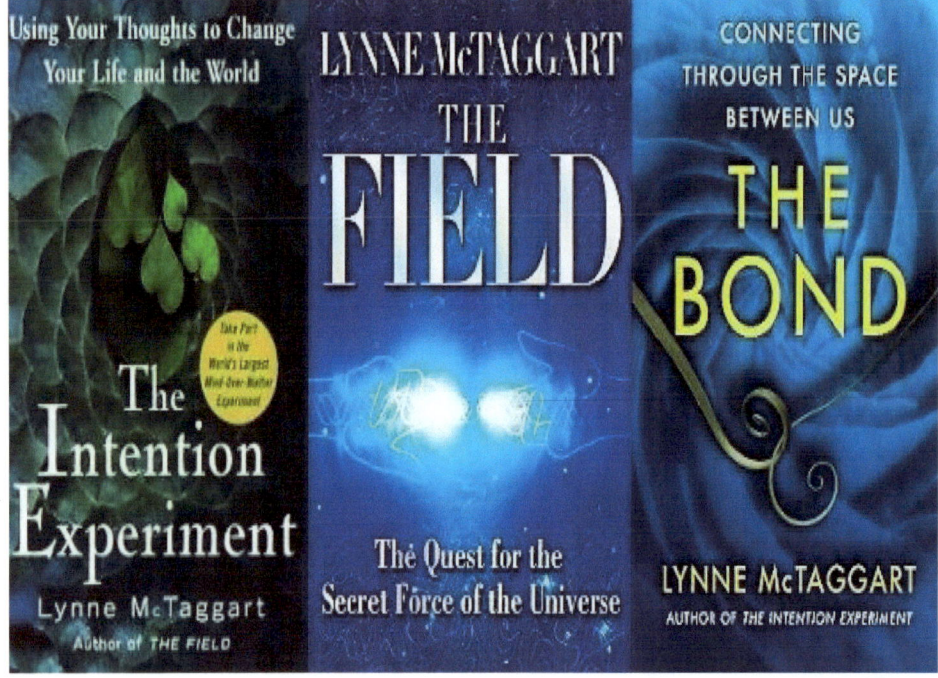

Using Your Thoughts to Change Your Life and the World

The Intention Experiment

Lynne McTaggart

Author of *THE FIELD*

LYNNE McTAGGART

THE FIELD

The Quest for the Secret Force of the Universe

CONNECTING THROUGH THE SPACE BETWEEN US

THE BOND

LYNNE McTAGGART

AUTHOR OF *THE INTENTION EXPERIMENT*

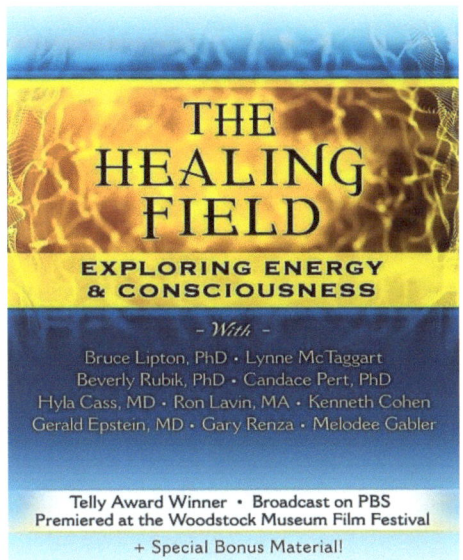

THE HEALING FIELD

EXPLORING ENERGY & CONSCIOUSNESS

– With –

Bruce Lipton, PhD • Lynne McTaggart
Beverly Rubik, PhD • Candace Pert, PhD
Hyla Cass, MD • Ron Lavin, MA • Kenneth Cohen
Gerald Epstein, MD • Gary Renza • Melodee Gabler

Telly Award Winner • Broadcast on PBS
Premiered at the Woodstock Museum Film Festival

+ Special Bonus Material!

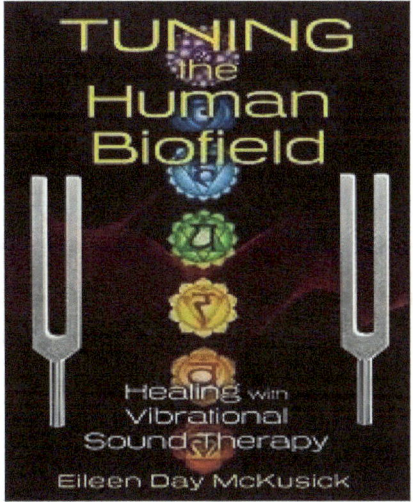

TUNING the Human Biofield

Healing with Vibrational Sound Therapy

Eileen Day McKusick

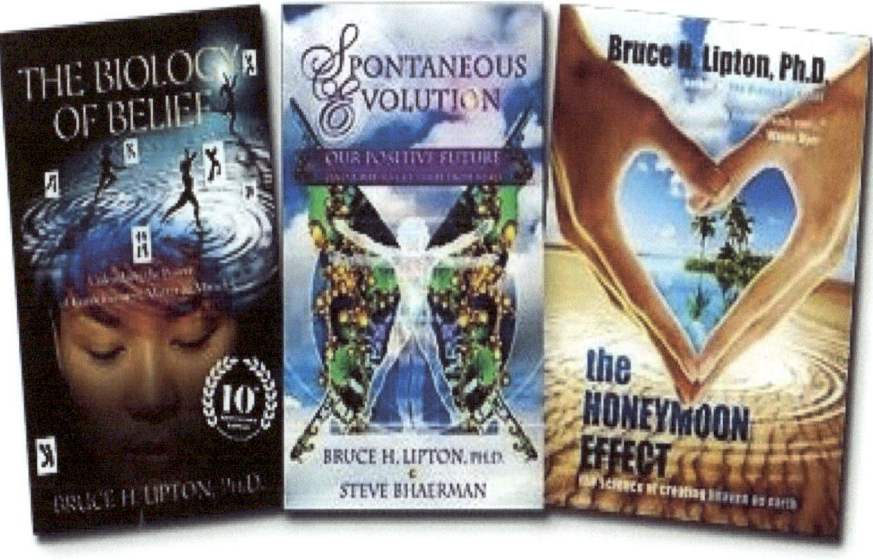

THE BIOLOGY OF BELIEF

BRUCE H. LIPTON, Ph.D.

Spontaneous Evolution

OUR POSITIVE FUTURE

BRUCE H. LIPTON, Ph.D.
& STEVE BHAERMAN

Bruce H. Lipton, Ph.D.

the HONEYMOON EFFECT

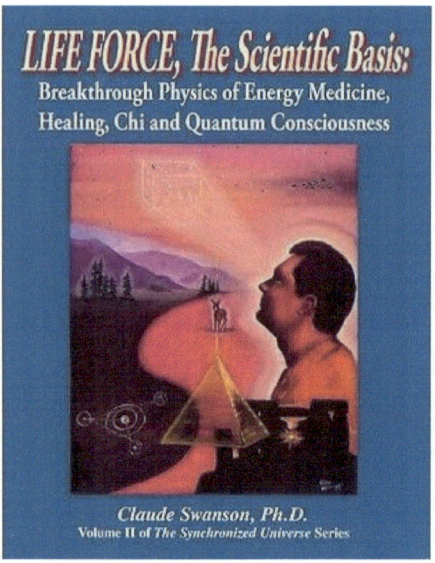

LIFE FORCE, The Scientific Basis:
Breakthrough Physics of Energy Medicine, Healing, Chi and Quantum Consciousness
Claude Swanson, Ph.D.
Volume II of *The Synchronized Universe* Series

Thank you, brother Ra Min for sharing these three books.

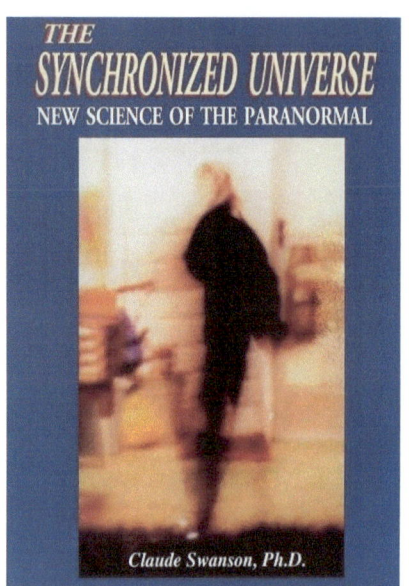

THE SYNCHRONIZED UNIVERSE
NEW SCIENCE OF THE PARANORMAL
Claude Swanson, Ph.D.

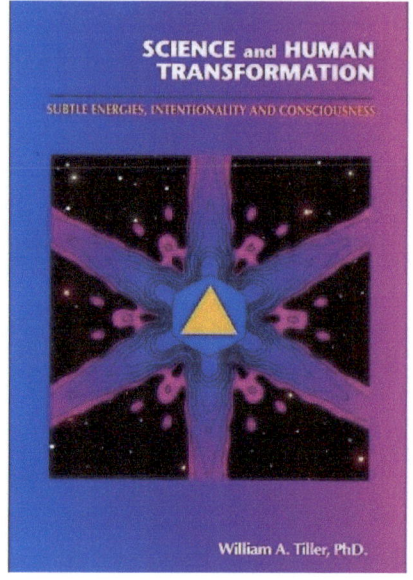

SCIENCE and HUMAN TRANSFORMATION
SUBTLE ENERGIES, INTENTIONALITY AND CONSCIOUSNESS
William A. Tiller, PhD.

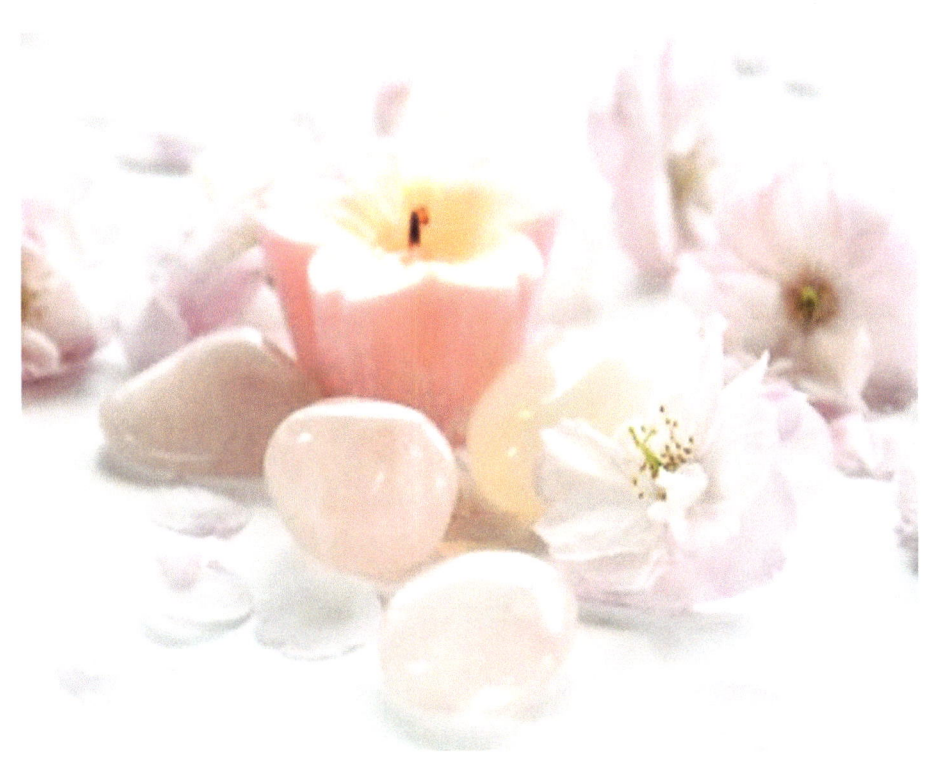

Heal On

Here are some healing modalities/energy healing tools from around the world!

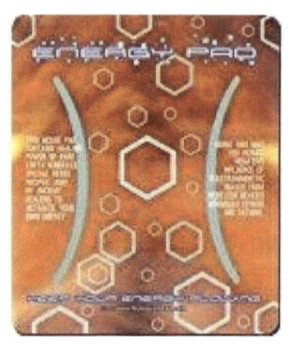

ENERGY PAD Natural Energy Activator, Resonance Therapy Device.

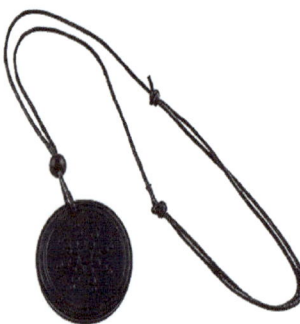

EHM Energy Balance Pendant - Negative Ion Balance Power - Improved Effect & Benefits Volcanic Lava Nano-Fusion Charm - Electromagnetic Field Protection & Energy Biofield Treatment Aid.

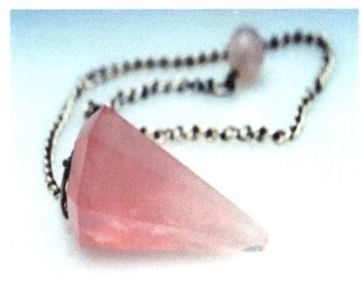
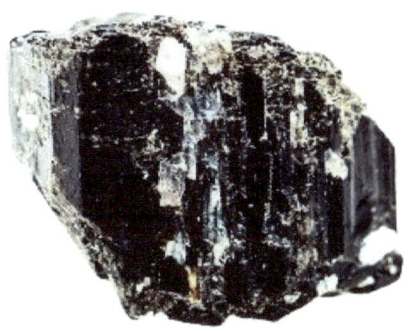

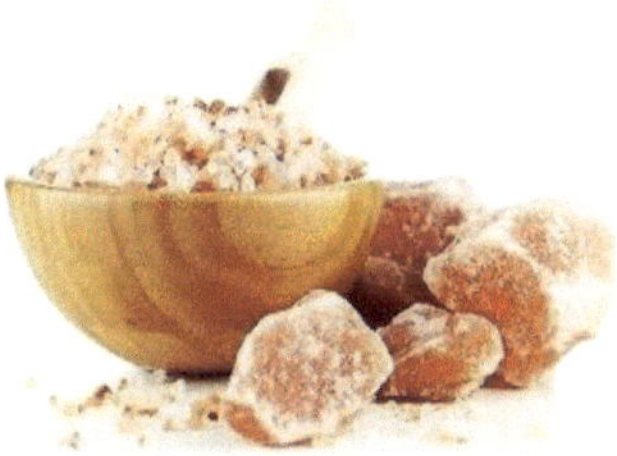

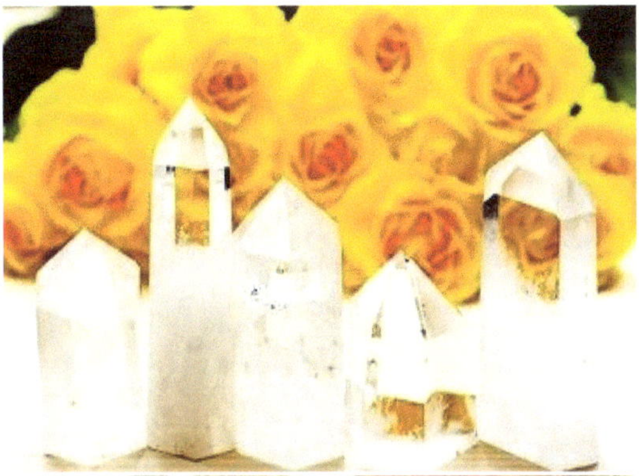

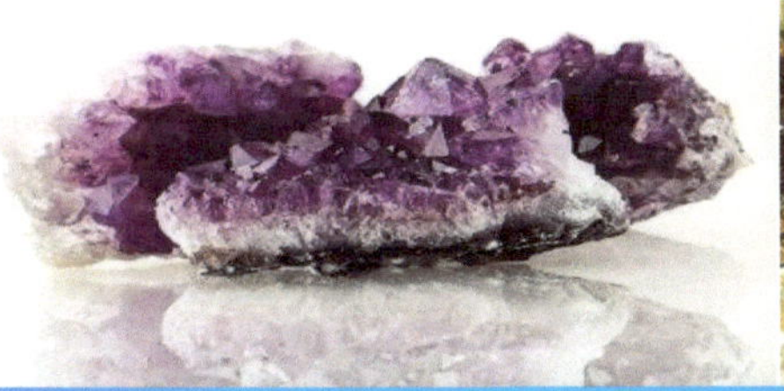

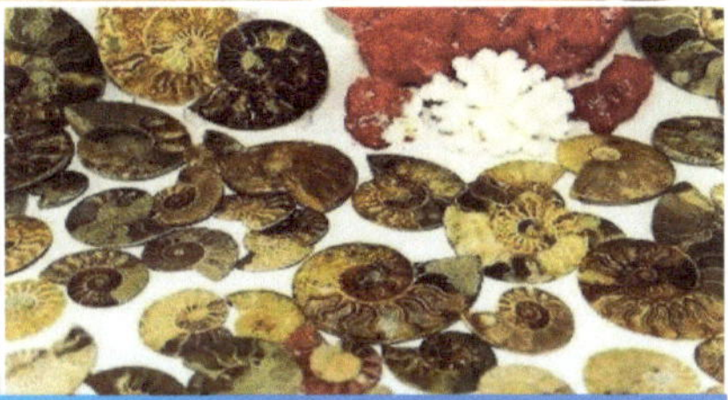

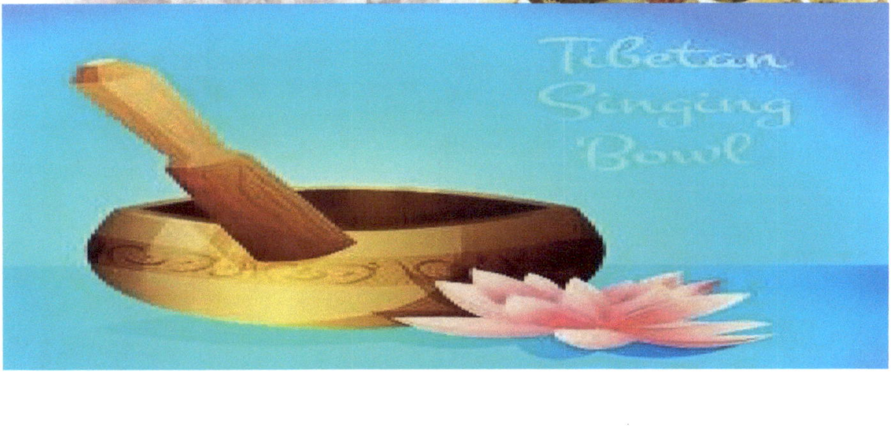

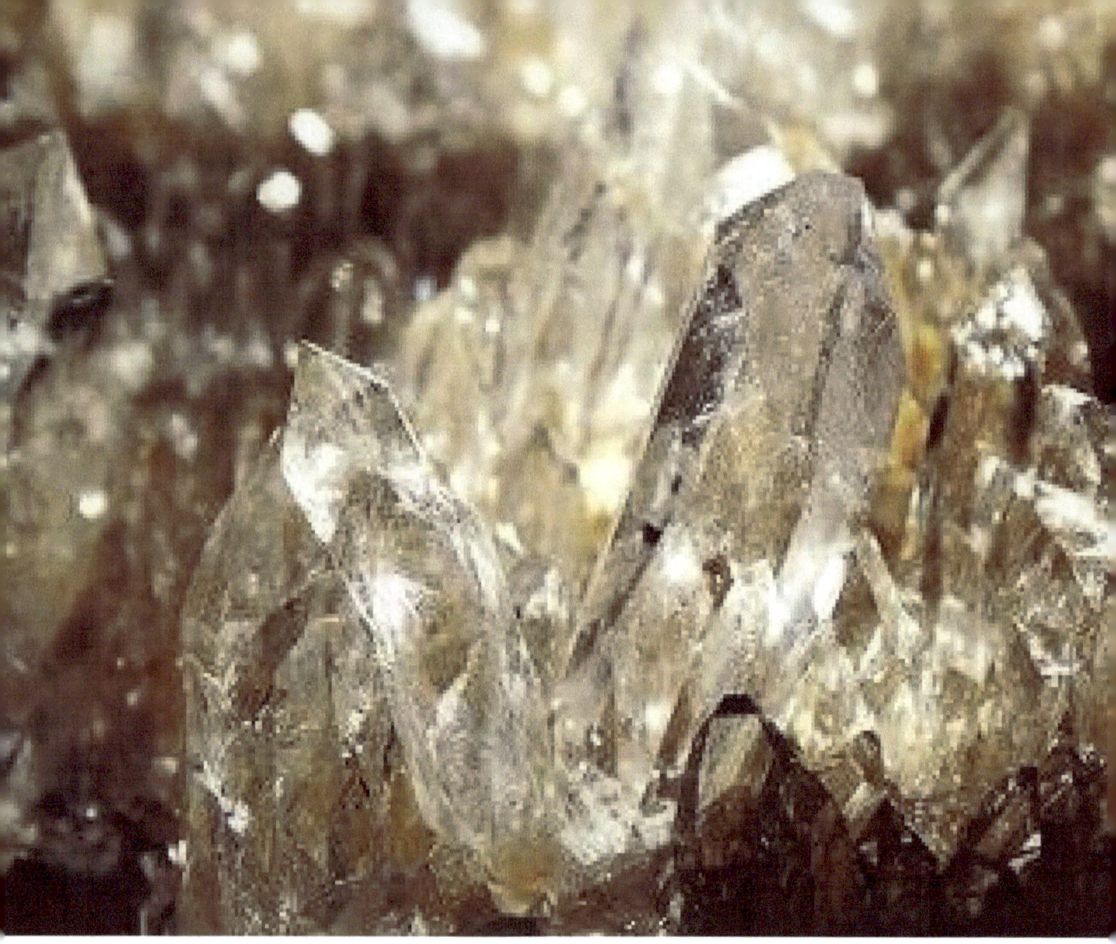

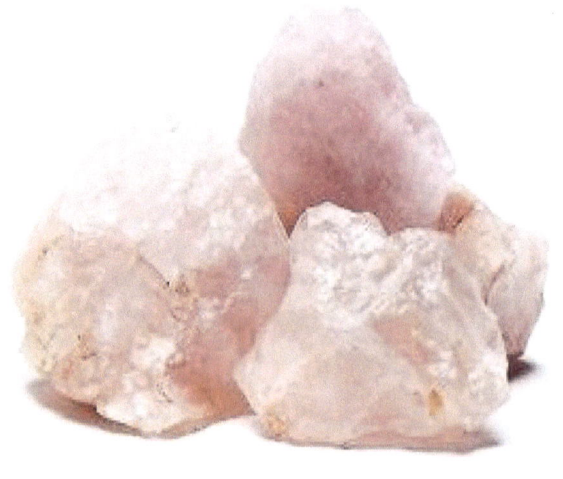

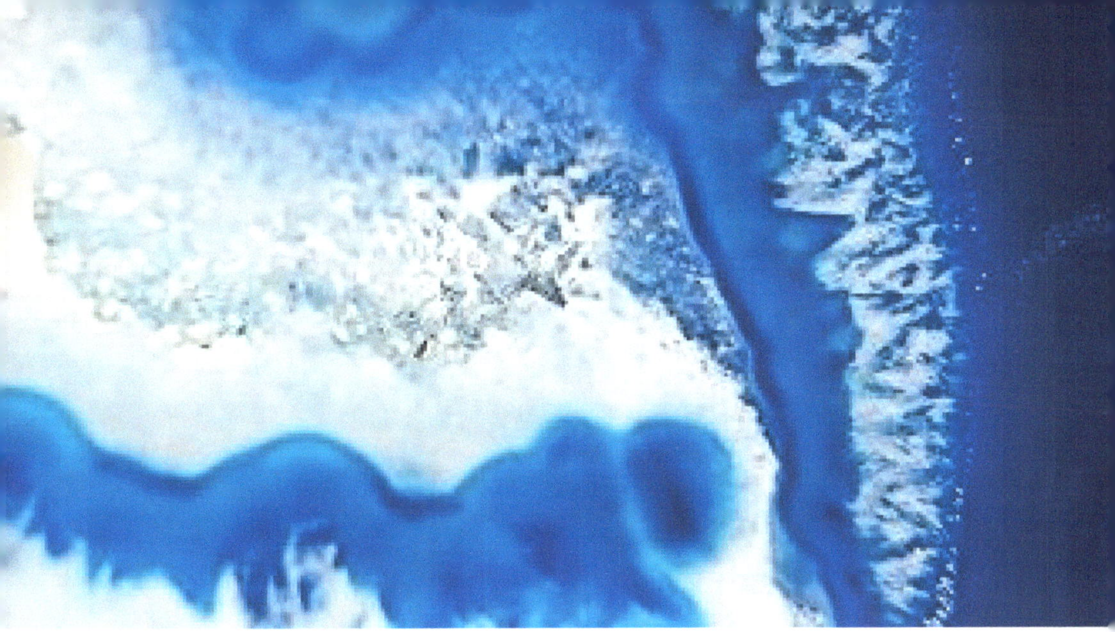

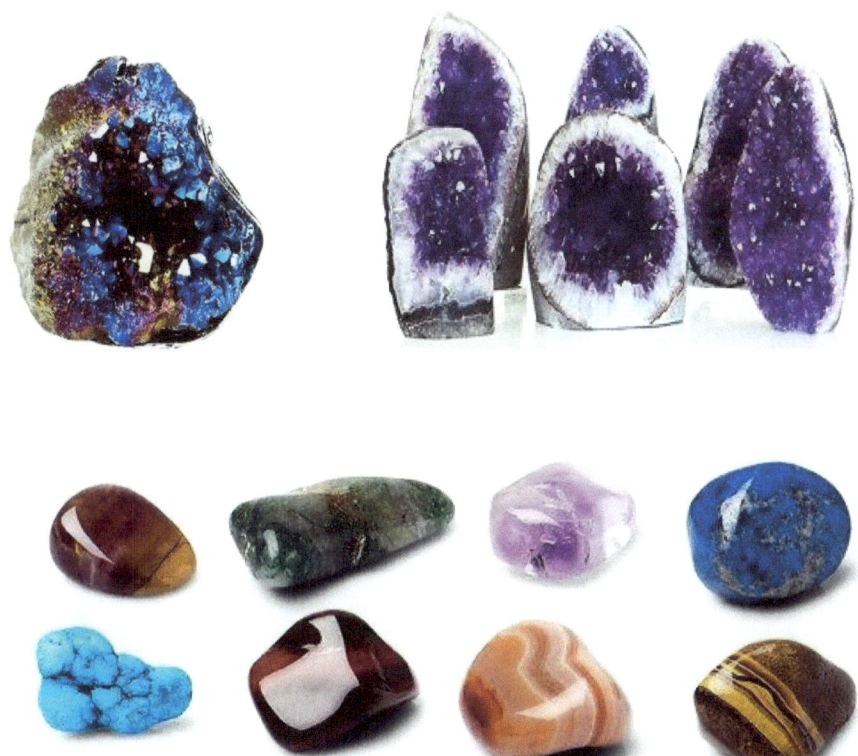

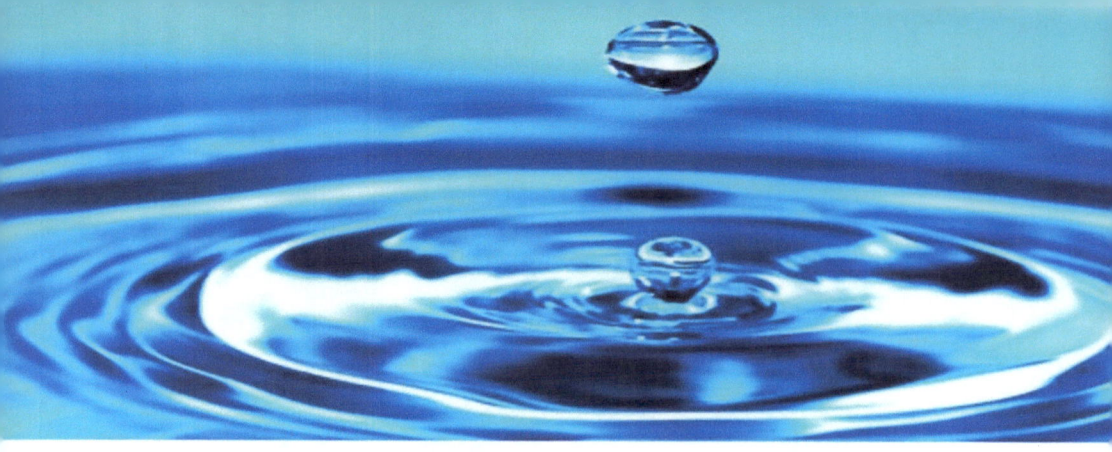

The human body contain about 70-90 percent of water.

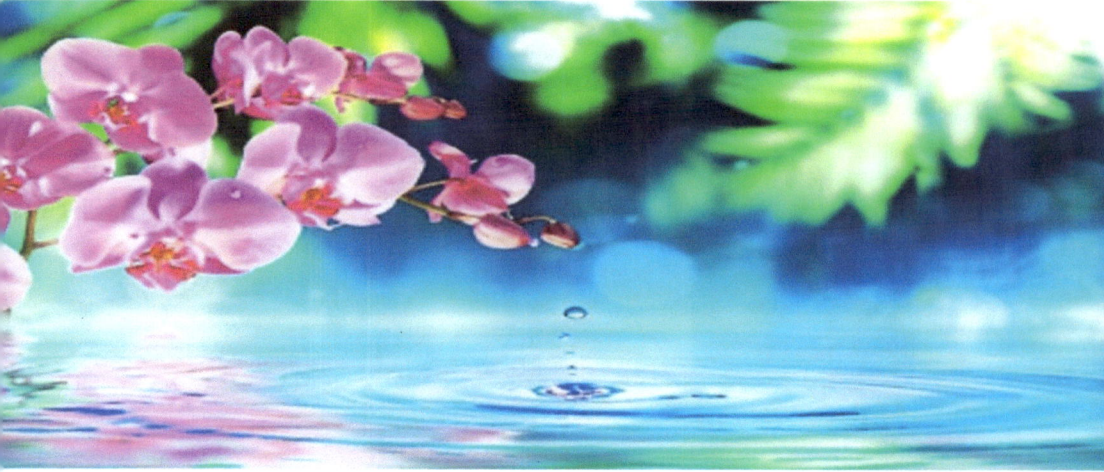

Water has memory. It can record and store information!

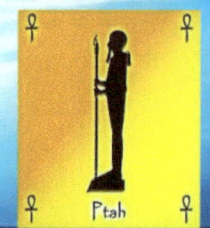

Everything is a wave.

Ptah, the molder. Mold
your water. Mold thyself;
to a higher frequency.

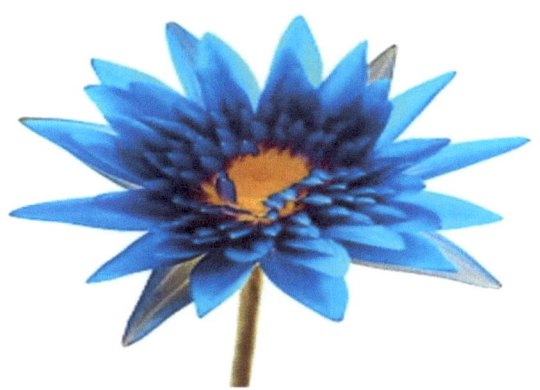

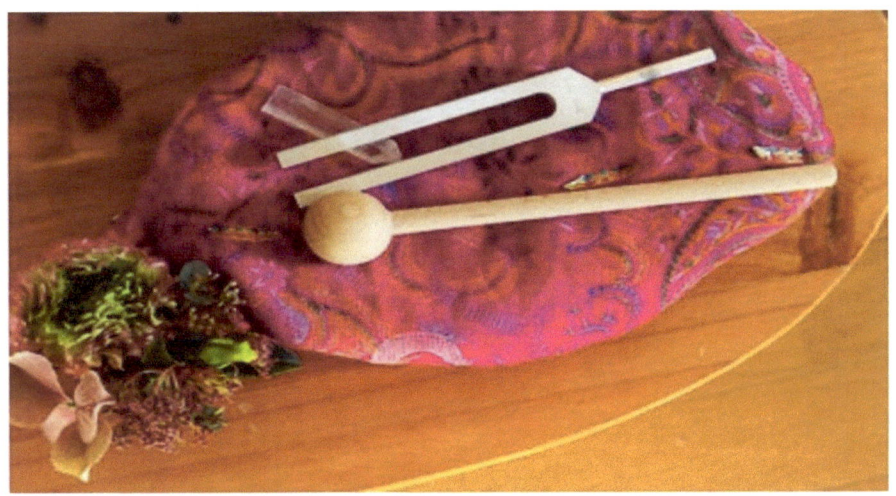

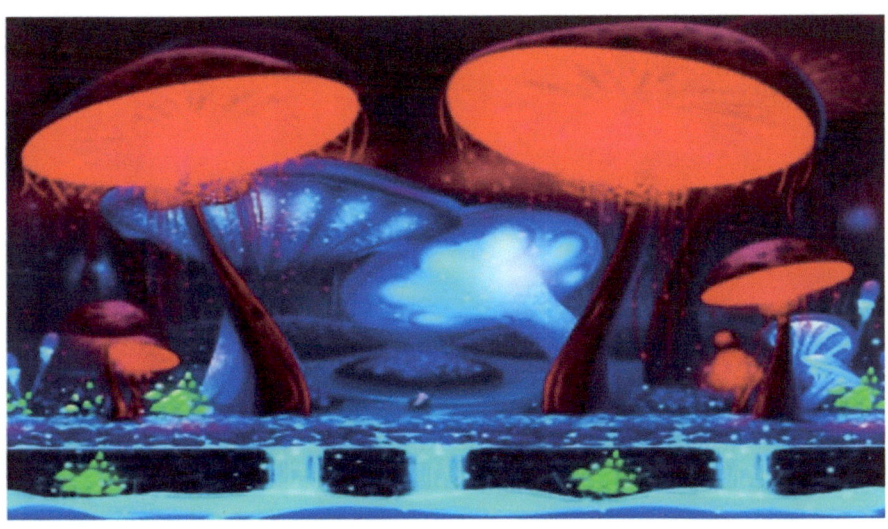

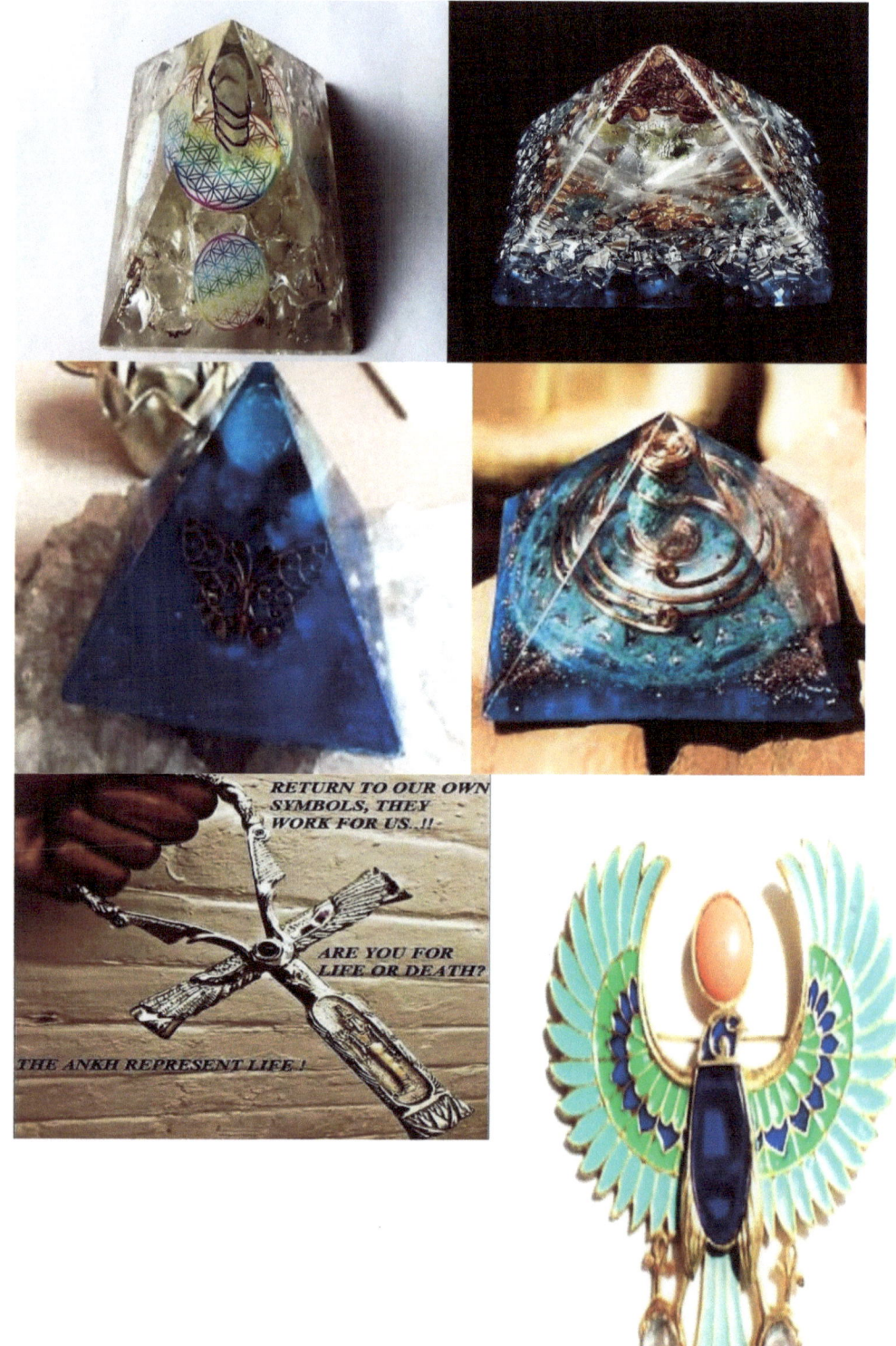

RETURN TO OUR OWN SYMBOLS, THEY WORK FOR US..!!

ARE YOU FOR LIFE OR DEATH?

THE ANKH REPRESENT LIFE !

Ancient day Africans are the parents of humanity. They taught the world.

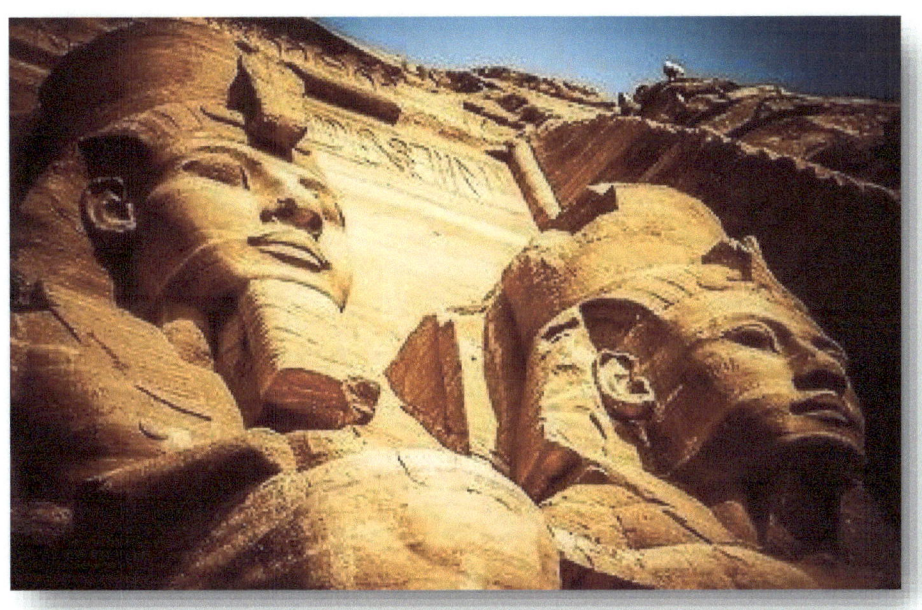

They live in us. Their Spirits are very much alive! Their works are here for us to see and learn from.

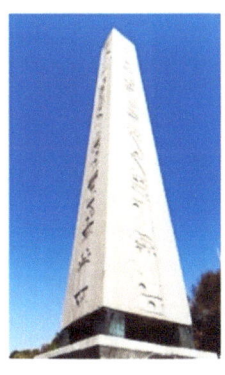

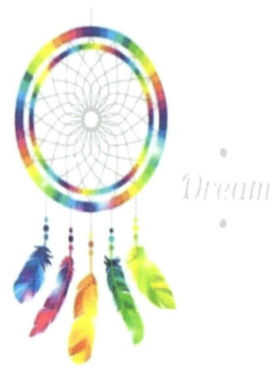

Dream

Indigenous/Native
American Healing

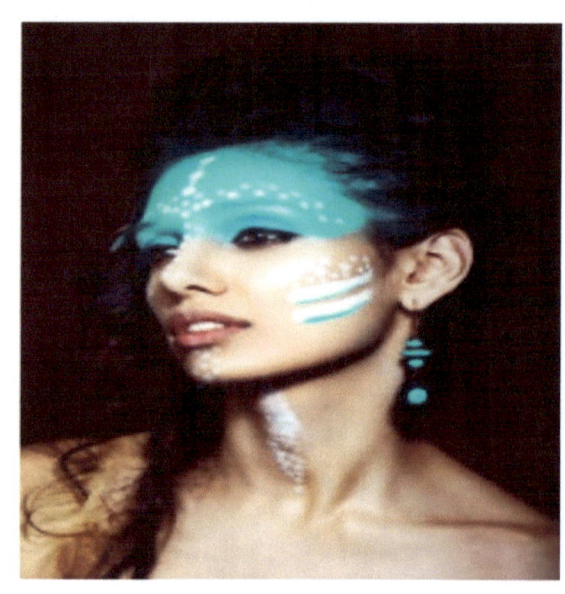

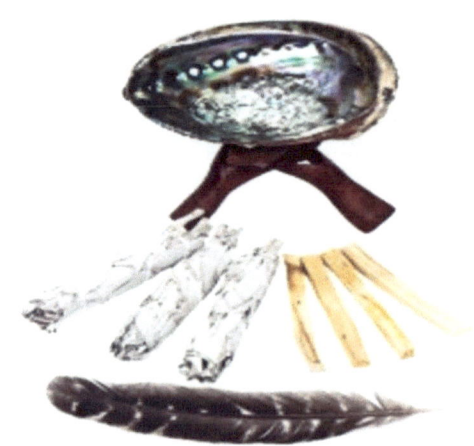

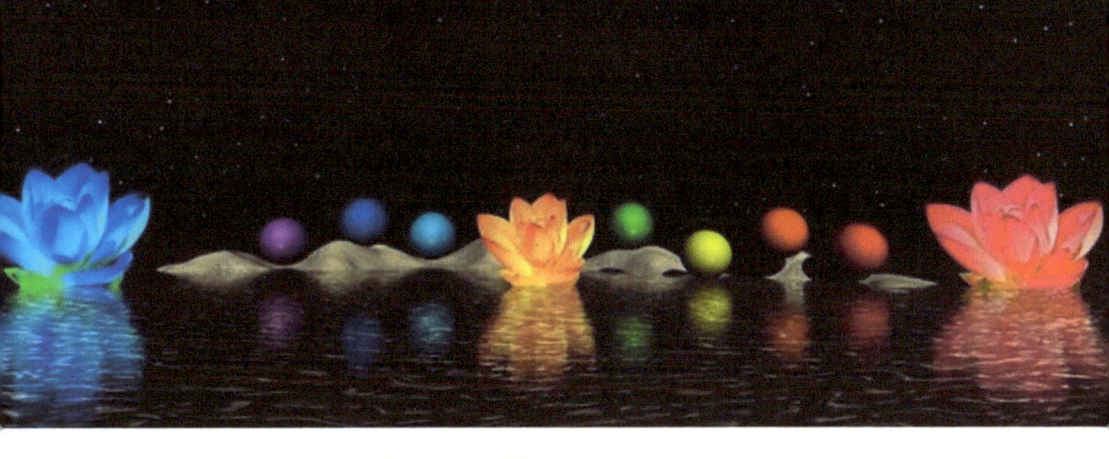

Asian Healing

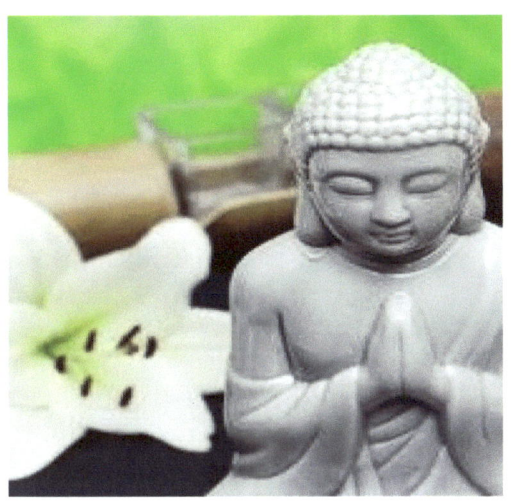

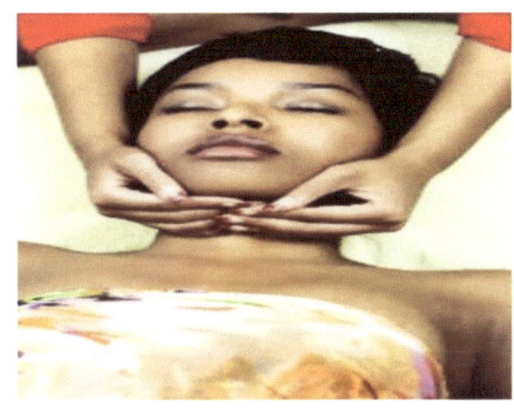

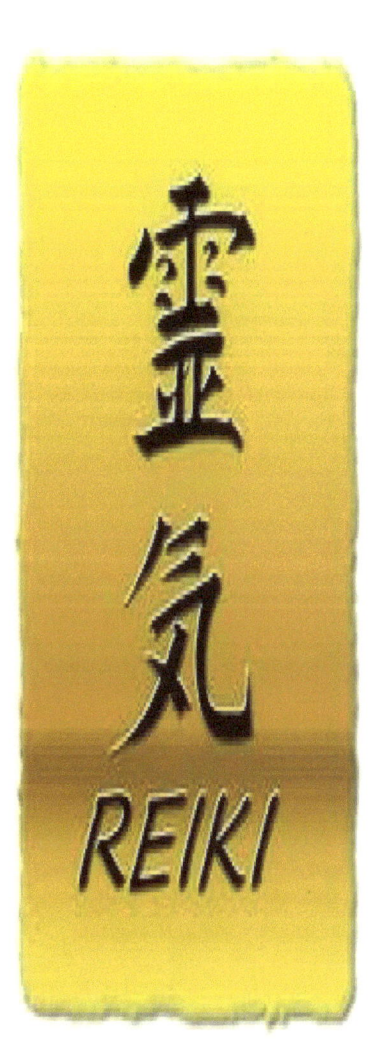

霊

気

REIKI

More Healing

Foot Reflexology Chart

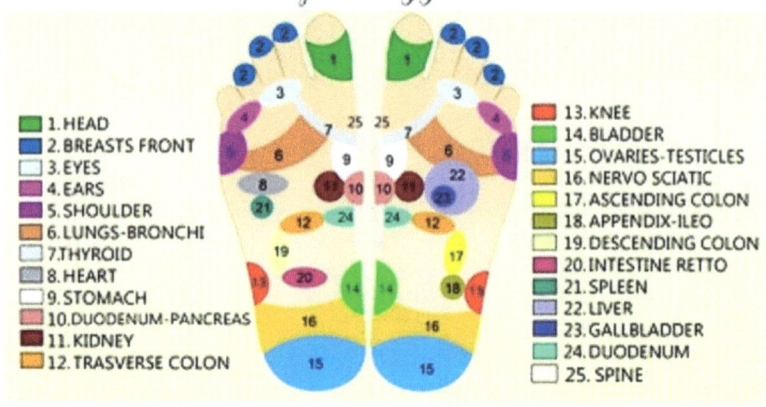

1. HEAD
2. BREASTS FRONT
3. EYES
4. EARS
5. SHOULDER
6. LUNGS-BRONCHI
7. THYROID
8. HEART
9. STOMACH
10. DUODENUM-PANCREAS
11. KIDNEY
12. TRASVERSE COLON
13. KNEE
14. BLADDER
15. OVARIES-TESTICLES
16. NERVO SCIATIC
17. ASCENDING COLON
18. APPENDIX-ILEO
19. DESCENDING COLON
20. INTESTINE RETTO
21. SPLEEN
22. LIVER
23. GALLBLADDER
24. DUODENUM
25. SPINE

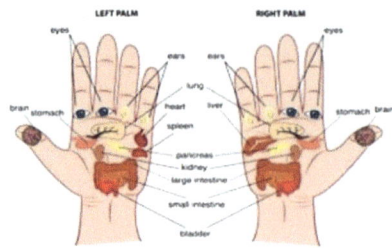

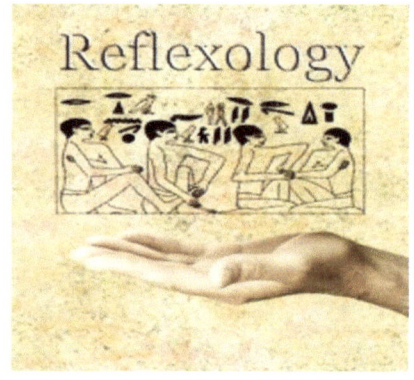

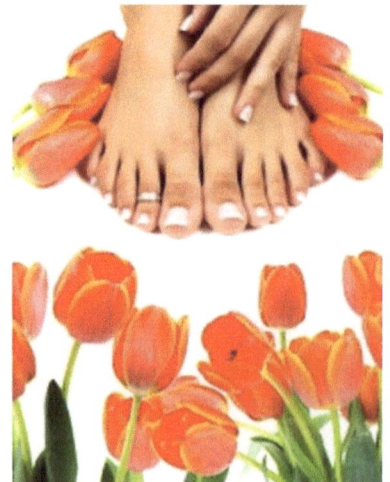

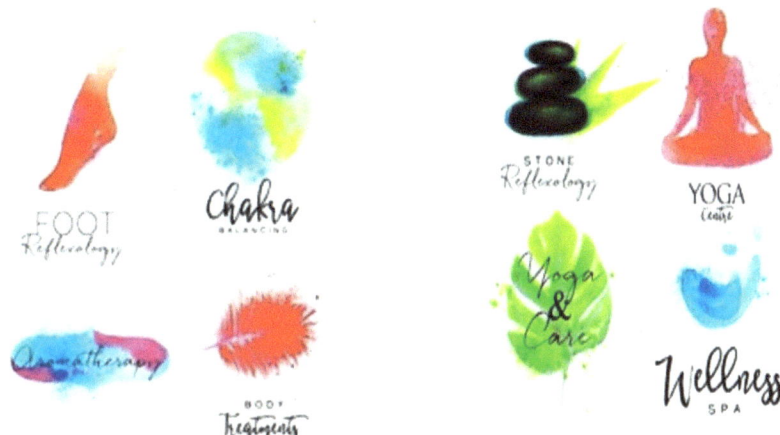

FOOT
Reflexology

Chakra
BALANCING

Aromatherapy

BODY
Treatments

STONE
Reflexology

YOGA
Centre

Yoga
&
Care

Wellness
SPA

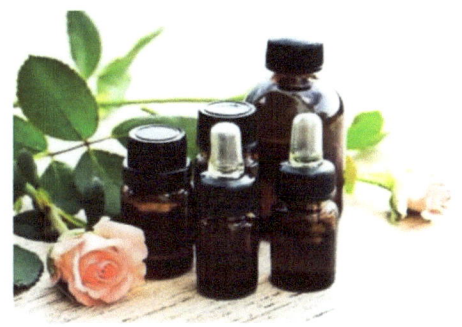

Oils

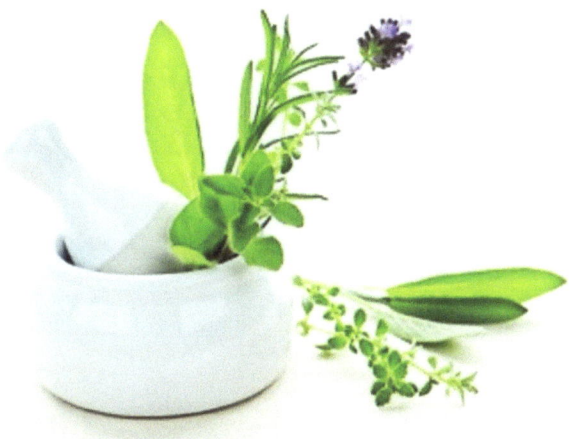

Herbs

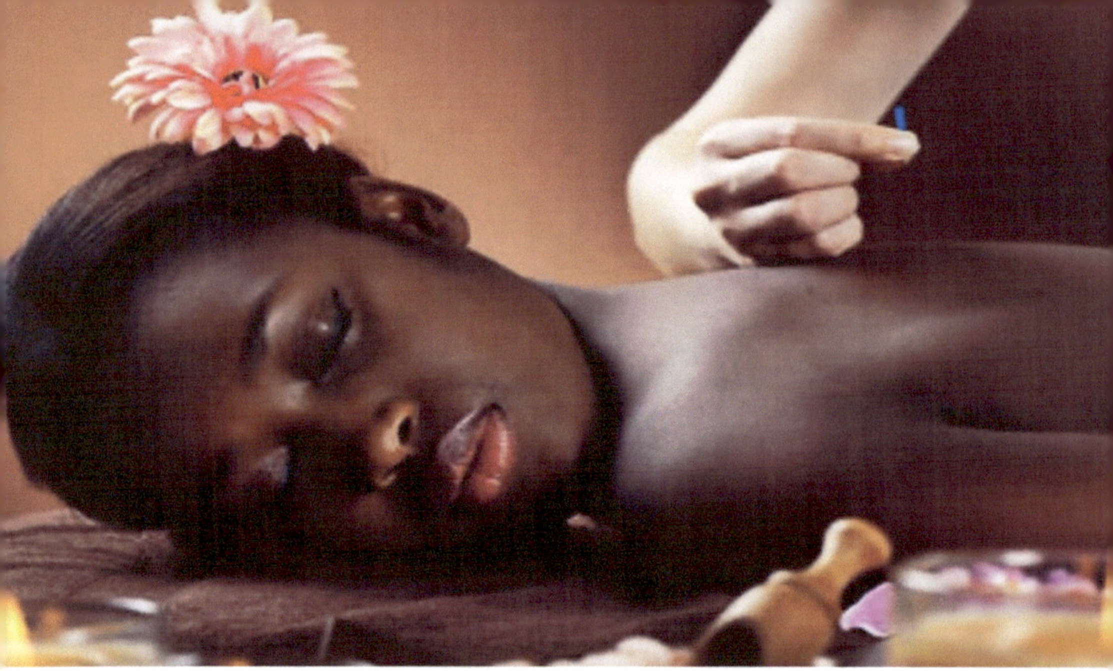

Acupuncture & Massage

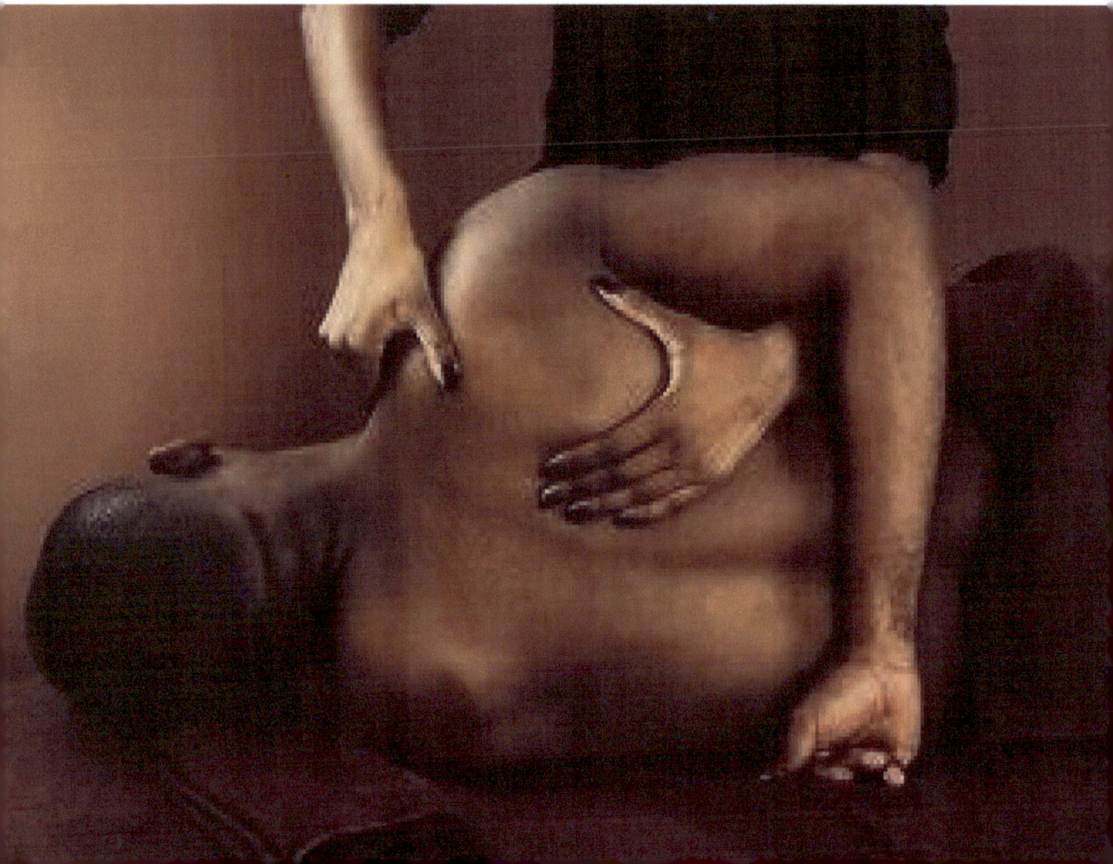

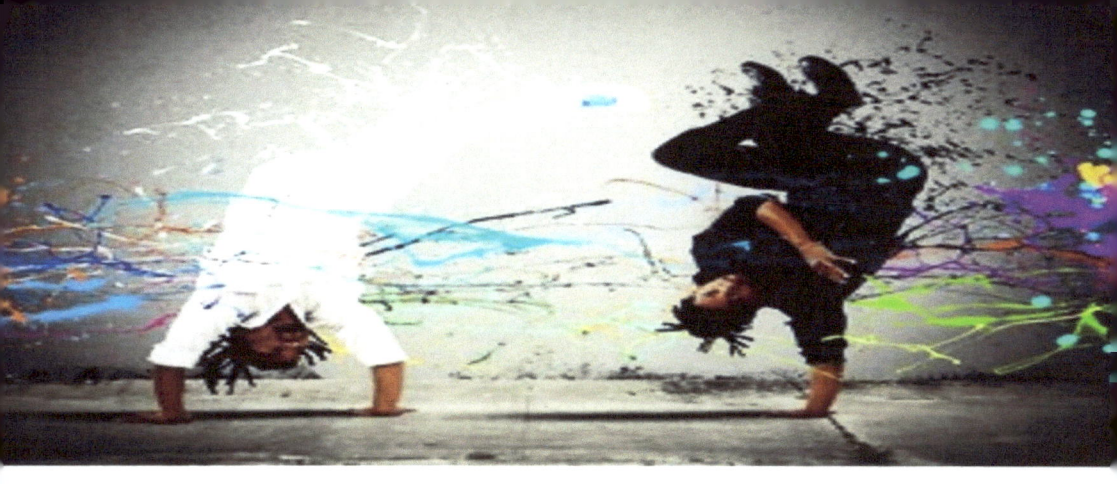

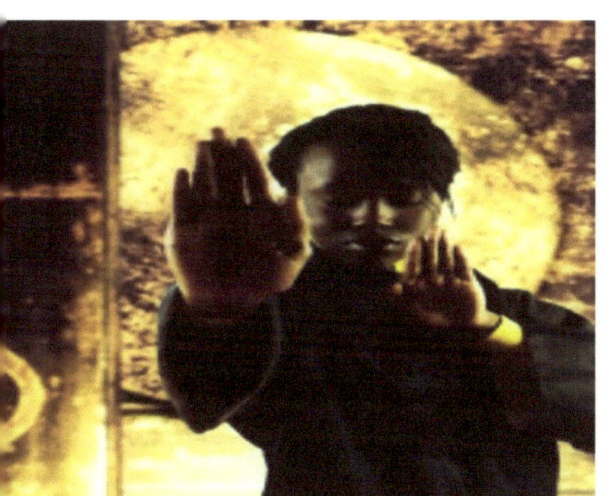

Martial Arts

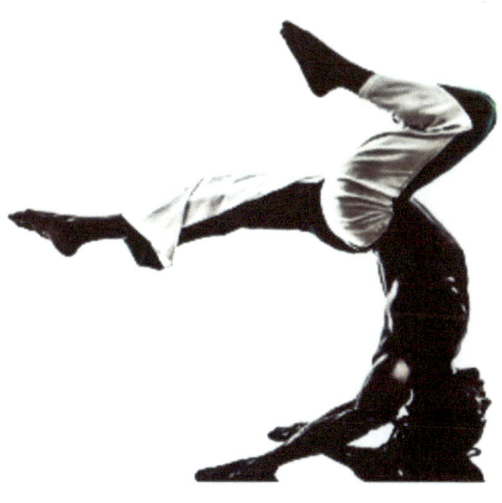

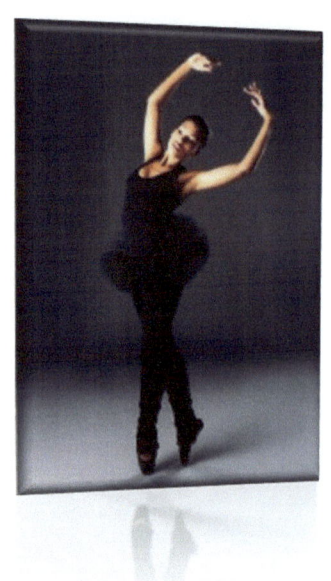

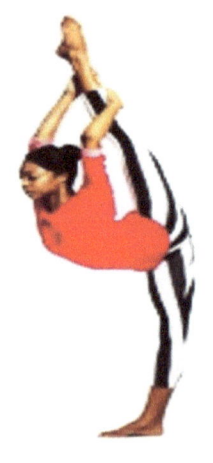

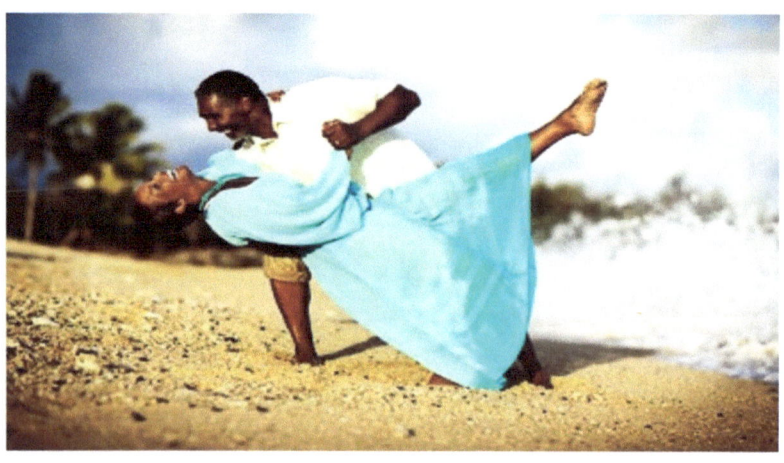

Dance

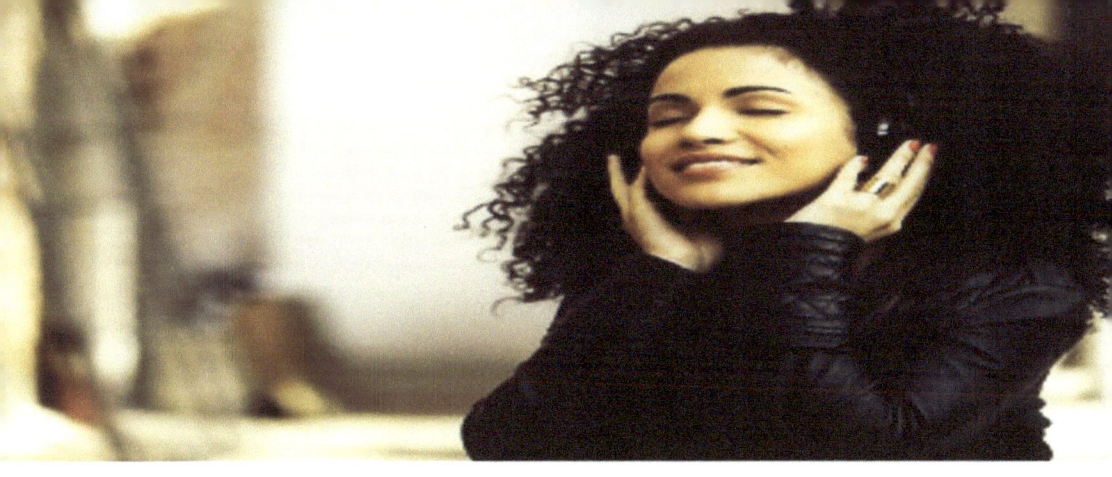

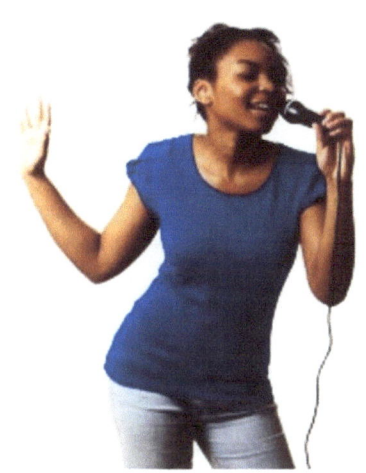

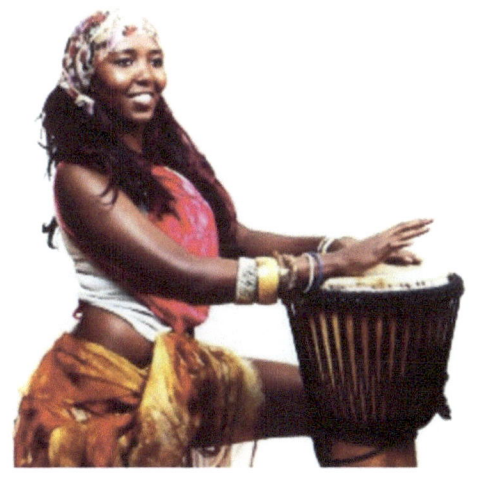

Music

Laughther Brings Forth Healing

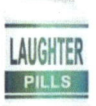

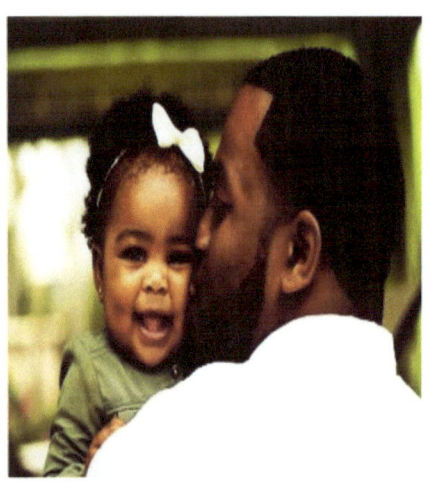

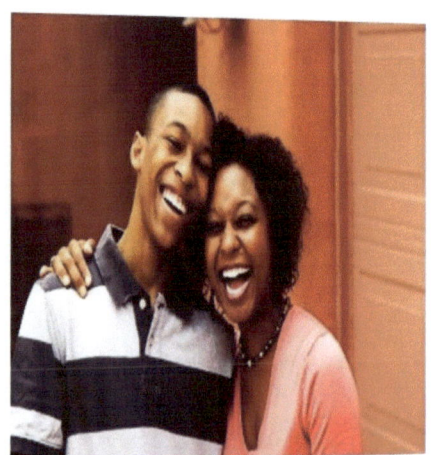

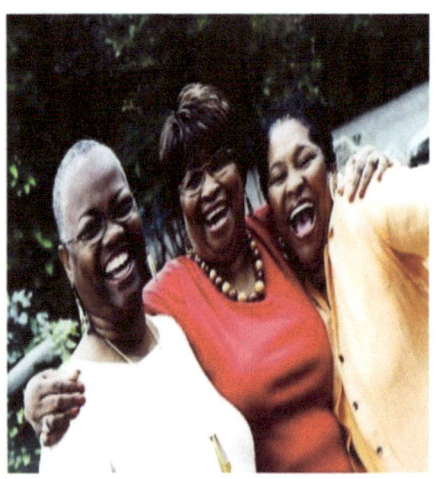

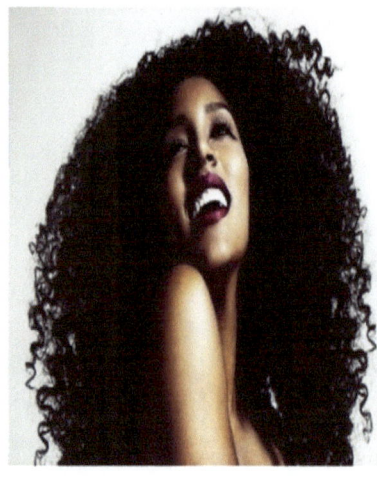

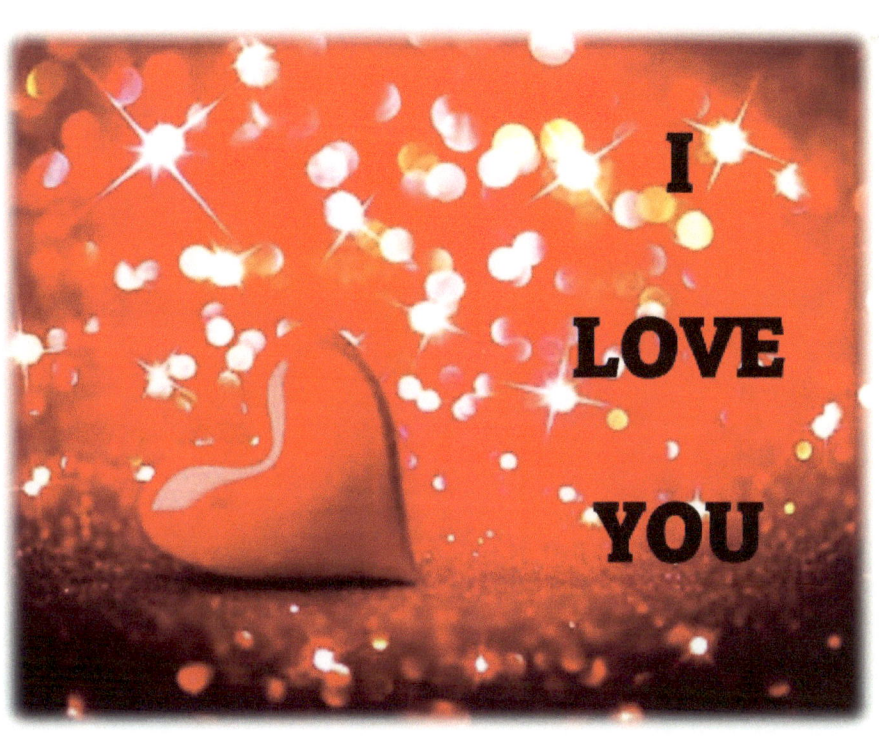

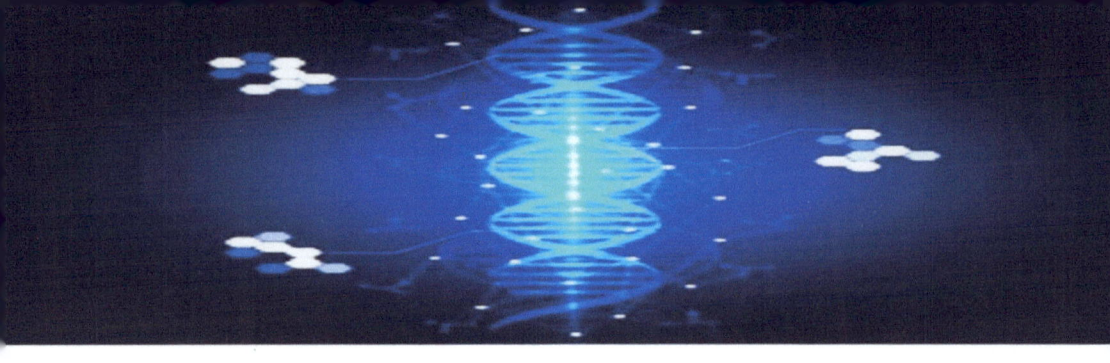

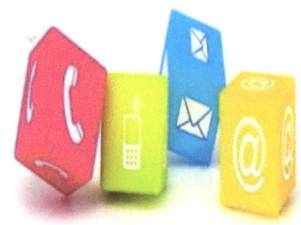

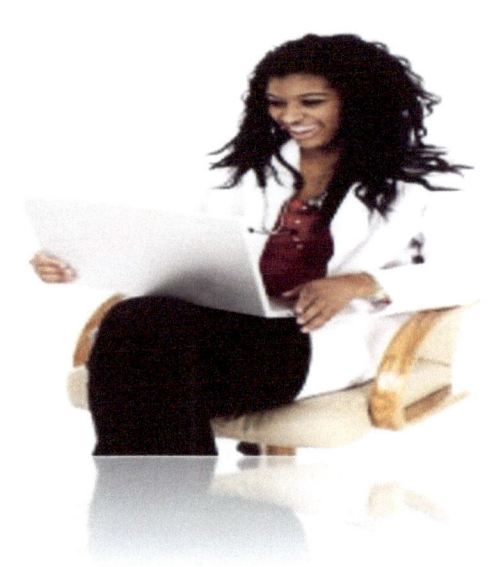

Contact:

HetHeru AnkhBaRa

718.314.4492

healingbluelotus.com

healingbluelotus@gmail.com

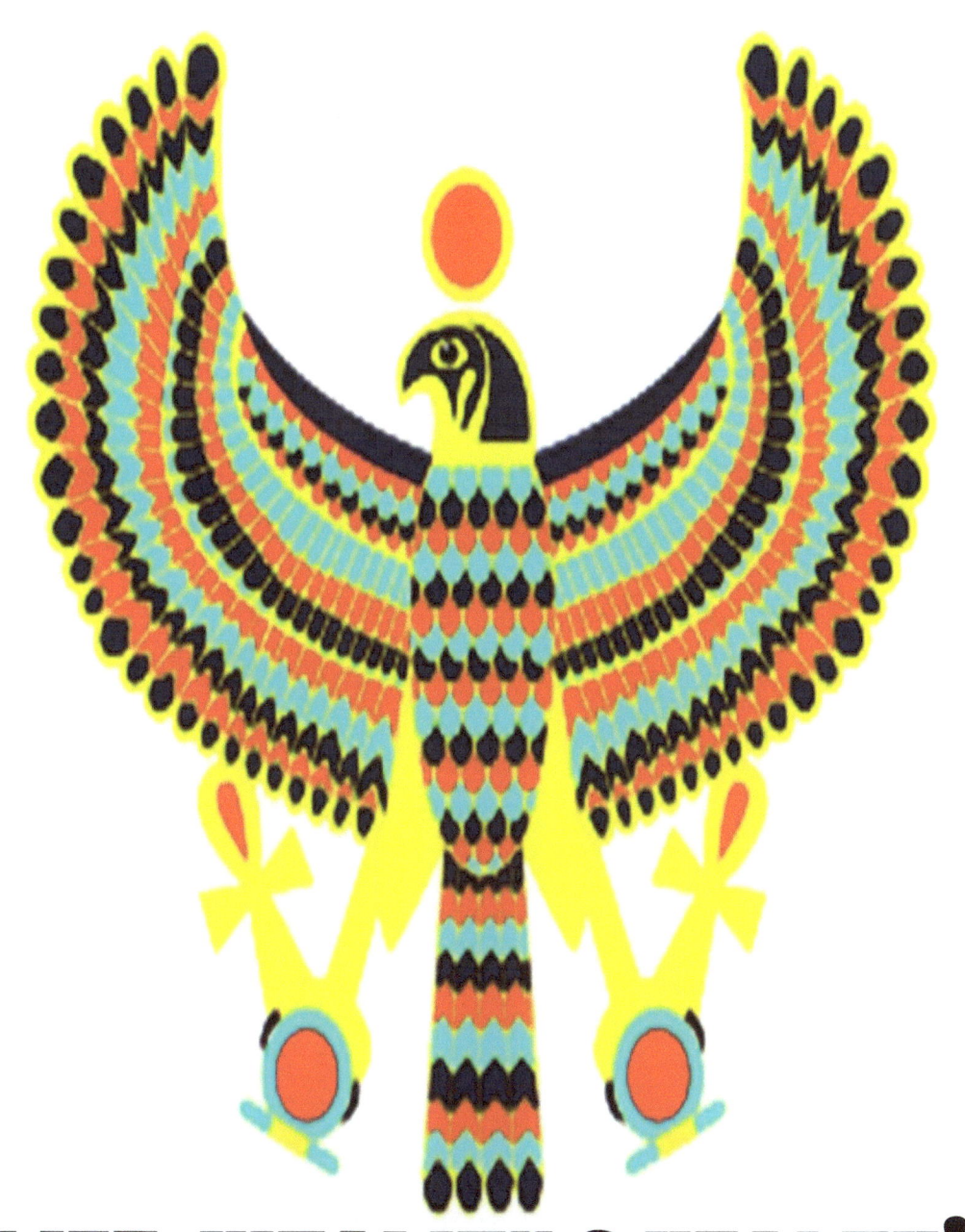

LIFE, VITALITY & HEALTH!

www.ingramcontent.com/pod-product-compliance
Lightning Source LLC
Chambersburg PA
CBHW040312010626
45792CB00022B/180